Praise for
The Glucose Revolution, The Glucose Revolution Life Plan and The Glucose Revolution Pocket Guides

■

"The concept of the glycemic index has been distorted and bastardized by popular writers and diet gurus. Here, at last, is a book that explains what we know about the glycemic index and its importance in designing a diet for optimum health. Carbohydrates are not all bad. Read the good news about pasta and even—believe it or not—sugar!"
—ANDREW WEIL, M.D., University of Arizona College of Medicine, author of *Spontaneous Healing* and *8 Weeks to Optimum Health*

■

"Forget *Sugar Busters*. Forget *The Zone*. If you want the real scoop on how carbohydrates and sugar affect your body, read this book by the world's leading researchers on the subject. It's the authoritative, last word on choosing foods to control your blood sugar."
—JEAN CARPER, best-selling author of *Miracle Cures, Stop Aging Now!* and *Food: Your Miracle Medicine*

■

"Mounting evidence indicates that refined carbohydrates and high glycemic index foods are contributing to the escalating epidemics of obesity and type 2 diabetes worldwide. This dietary pattern also appears to increase the risk of heart disease and stroke. The skyrocketing proportion of calories from added sugars and refined carbohydrates in westernized diets portends a future acceleration of these trends. *The Glucose Revolution* challenges traditional doctrines about optimal nutrition and the role of carbohydrates in health and disease. Brand-Miller and colleagues are to be congratulated for an eminently lucid and important book that explains the science behind the glycemic index and provides tools and strategies for modifying diet to incorporate this knowledge. I strongly recommend the book to both health professionals and the general public who could use this state-of-the-art information to improve health and well-being."

—JOANN E. MANSON, M.D., D.P.H.,
Professor of Medicine, Harvard Medical School,
and Co-Director of Women's Health, Division of
Preventive Medicine, Brigham and Women's Hospital

∎

"Here is at last a book explaining the importance of taking into consideration the glycemic index of foods for overall health, athletic performance, and in reducing the risk of heart disease and diabetes. The book clearly explains that there are different kinds of carbohydrates that work in different ways and why a universal recommendation to 'increase the carbohydrate content of your diet' is plainly simple and scientifically inaccurate. Everyone should put the glycemic index approach into practice."

—ARTEMIS P. SIMOPOULOS, M.D.,
senior author of *The Omega Diet* and
The Healing Diet and President, The Center for
Genetics, Nutrition and Health, Washington, D.C.

"*The Glucose Revolution* is nutrition science for the 21st century. Clearly written, it gives the scientific rationale for why all carbohydrates are not created equal. It is a practical guide for both professionals and patients. The food suggestions and recipes are exciting and tasty."

—RICHARD N. PODELL, M.D., M.P.H.,
Clinical Professor, Department of Family Medicine,
UMDNJ–Robert Wood Johnson Medical School,
and coauthor of *The G-Index Diet: The Missing Link That Makes Permanent Weight Loss Possible*

"Although the jury is still out on the utility of the glycemic index, many of the curious will benefit from a careful reading of this book, and some will find that the glycemic index is particularly helpful for them. Everyone can enjoy the recipes, some of which are to die for!"

—JOHANNA DWYER, D.Sc., R.D.,
editor of *Nutrition Today*

The Glucose Revolution Pocket Guide to
THE GLYCEMIC INDEX AND HEALTHY KIDS

OTHER *GLUCOSE REVOLUTION* TITLES

The Glucose Revolution: The Authoritative Guide to the Glycemic Index—The Groundbreaking Medical Discovery

The Glucose Revolution Life Plan

■

The Glucose Revolution Pocket Guide to the Top 100 Low Glycemic Foods

The Glucose Revolution Pocket Guide to Diabetes

The Glucose Revolution Pocket Guide to Losing Weight

The Glucose Revolution Pocket Guide to Sports Nutrition

The Glucose Revolution Pocket Guide to Sugar and Energy

The Glucose Revolution Pocket Guide to Your Heart

The Glucose Revolution Pocket Guide to Children with Type 1 Diabetes

The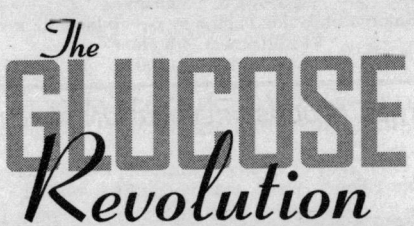

POCKET GUIDE TO
THE GLYCEMIC INDEX AND HEALTHY KIDS

HEATHER GILBERTSON,
B. SC., GRAD. DIP. DIET., GRAD. CERT. DIAB. ED., APD
JENNIE BRAND-MILLER, PH.D.
KAYE FOSTER-POWELL, B.SC., M. NUTR. & DIET.
THOMAS M.S. WOLEVER, M.D., PH.D.

ADAPTED BY
JOHANNA BURANI, M.S., R.D., C.D.E.,
AND LINDA RAO, M.ED.

■

MARLOWE & COMPANY
NEW YORK

Published by
Marlowe & Company
An Imprint of Avalon Publishing Group Incorporated
841 Broadway, 4th Floor
New York, NY 10003

THE GLUCOSE REVOLUTION POCKET GUIDE TO THE
GLYCEMIC INDEX AND HEALTHY KIDS

Copyright © 2000, 2001 by Heather Gilbertson, Dr. Jennie Brand-Miller,
Kaye Foster-Powell, and Thomas M.S. Wolever

All rights reserved. No part of this book may be reproduced in whole or in part without written permission from the publisher, except by reviewers who may quote brief excerpts in connection with a review in a newspaper, magazine, or electronic publication; nor may any part of this book be reproduced, stored in a retrieval system, or transmitted in any form or by any means, electronic, mechanical, photocopying, recording, or other, without written permission from the publisher.

The information in this book is intended to help readers make informed decisions about their health and the health of their loved ones. It is not intended to be a substitute for treatment by or the advice and care of a professional health care provider. While the authors and publisher have endeavored to ensure that the information is accurate and up to date, they are not responsible for adverse effects or consequences sustained by any person using this book.

First published in Australia in 2000 under the title *The Glucose Revolution G.I. Plus Pocket Guide to the G.I. Factor for Healthy Kids* by Hodder Headline Australia Pty Limited.

This edition is published by arrangement with
Hodder Headline Pty Limited

Library of Congress Cataloging-in-Publication Data

Brand-Miller, Janette, 1952-
  The glucose revolution pocket guide to the glycemic index and
  healthy kids / by Jennie Brand-Miller, Kaye Foster-Powell, and
Thomas M.S. Wolever.
    p. cm.
  ISBN 1-56924-588-6
  1. Children—Nutrition. 2. Glycemic index. 3. Sugar—Health
aspects 4. High-carbohydrate diet. 5. Carbohydrates in human
nutrition. I. Title: Foster-Powell, Kaye. II. Wolever, Thomas M.S.
III. Title.

RJ206 .B73 2001
612.3'96'083—dc21

2001030144

9 8 7 6 5 4 3 2 1

Designed by Pauline Neuwirth, Neuwirth & Associates, Inc.
Distributed by Publishers Group West
Manufactured in the United States of America

CONTENTS

Preface ... xi

1. How to Use This Book ... 1
2. What Is the Glucose Revolution? ... 3
3. The Glycemic Index: Some Background ... 5
4. How We Measure the Glycemic Index ... 9
5. Who Benefits from Low G.I. Foods? ... 13
6. A Healthy Diet for Children ... 15
7. The Way Children Eat ... 17
8. Why Our Children Are at Risk ... 19
9. G.I. Values and Children's Weight ... 21
10. Why We Need More Carbohydrate ... 23
11. Sources of Carbohydrate ... 25
12. Low G.I. Diets for Children ... 29
13. Food Basics ... 31
14. Sugar 101 ... 40
15. Activity and Sports ... 45
16. Eat to Compete ... 48
17. Tips for Lower G.I. Meals ... 51
18. The Food Pyramid for Children ... 53
19. A Week of Low G.I. Menus ... 56
20. Snacks and Light Meals ... 62
21. Breakfast Basics ... 64
22. School Lunch! ... 67
23. The Late-Morning Blahs ... 71
24. What's for Dinner? ... 73
25. Desserts: A Low G.I. Finish ... 76

26. Take-Out Foods	78
27. Your Questions Answered	80
28. How to Use the G.I. Tables	87
29. The Glycemic Index Tables	89

For More Information	105
About the Authors	108
Acknowledgments	111

PREFACE

The Glucose Revolution and *The Glucose Revolution Life Plan* are the definitive, all-in-one guides to the glycemic index (G.I.). Now we have written this pocket guide to show you how the glycemic index relates to children and their eating habits. As we explain in our previous books, the glycemic index:

- is a proven guide to the true physiological effects foods—especially carbohydrates—have on blood sugar levels;
- provides an easy and effective way to eat a healthy diet and control fluctuations in blood sugar.

This book offers more in-depth information about how the glycemic index affects children than we had room to include in our other books. In this volume, we've included the questions that people most frequently ask about children's nutrition and many other extras.

We've written this book as a companion to *The Glucose Revolution* and *The Glucose Revolution Life Plan*, so in the event you haven't already consulted those books, please be sure to do so for a more comprehensive discussion of the glycemic index and all its uses.

Chapter 1

HOW TO USE THIS BOOK

This pocket guide will help you to understand the glucose revolution and how you can use it to help your children grow up healthy, strong, and full of energy. After eating the low G.I. way, your children will be well on the road to a lifetime of healthy eating! In this book, we:

- explain which types of carbohydrate are best for children and why;
- show you how to include more of the right sort of carbohydrate in your children's diet;
- provide practical hints for meal preparation and tips to help make the G.I. work throughout the day;

- give you lots of low G.I. menus that children (even picky eaters) will love;
- include an A–Z listing of over 300 foods with their G.I. values and carbohydrate and fat grams.

Chapter 2

WHAT IS THE GLUCOSE REVOLUTION?

Our bodies burn fuel all the time. But for best performance we need the right type of fuel, and the energy source our bodies like best is carbohydrate. In fact, carbohydrates are our body's fuel of choice!

In our first book, *The Glucose Revolution*, we explained that not all carbohydrates are created equal, and we discussed how different types of carbohydrate work in different ways in our bodies. We revealed that some carbohydrates are absorbed much more slowly than others and that these slowly digested carbohydrates have startling health benefits for everybody. These carbohydrates:

- provide sustained energy;
- satisfy and reduce appetite;
- lower insulin levels, which makes you burn more—and store less—fat;
- help manage diabetes;
- reduce diabetes, heart disease, and certain cancer risks.

We also explained that eating the right *amount* of carbohydrate, as well as the right *type* of carbohydrate, makes a very important contribution to our quality of life, health and well being.

Our research has been described as a "glucose revolution" because it has turned many traditional beliefs about starchy foods upside down and has changed the way we think about carbohydrates forever!

Chapter 3

THE GLYCEMIC INDEX: SOME BACKGROUND

The glycemic index of foods is simply a ranking of foods based on their immediate effect on blood sugar levels. To make a fair comparison, all foods are compared with a reference food such as pure glucose and are tested in equivalent carbohydrate amounts.

Today we know the glycemic index of hundreds of different food items—both generic and namebrand—that have been tested following a standardized testing method. The tables on pages 90-103 give the glycemic index of a range of common foods, including many tested at the University of Toronto and the University of Sydney.

HOW THE GLYCEMIC INDEX CAME TO BE

The glycemic index concept was first developed in 1981 by a team of scientists led by Dr. David Jenkins, a professor of nutrition at the University of Toronto, Canada, to help determine which foods were best for people with diabetes. At that time, the diet for people with diabetes was based on a system of carbohydrate exchanges, or portions, that was complicated and not very logical. The carbohydrate exchange system assumed that all starchy foods produce the same effect on blood sugar levels, even though some earlier studies had already proven this was not correct. Jenkins was one of the first researchers to question this assumption and to investigate how real foods behave in the bodies of real people.

Jenkins's approach attracted a great deal of attention because it was so logical and systematic. He and his colleagues had tested a large number of common foods, and some of their results were surprising. Ice cream, for example, despite its sugar content, has much less effect on blood sugar than some ordinary breads. Over the next fifteen years medical researchers and scientists around the world, including the authors of this book, tested the effect of many foods on blood sugar levels and developed a new concept of classifying carbohydrates based on their glycemic index.

When we looked at the actual blood sugar responses to different foods in people we found that:

- many complex carbohydrates, such as bread and potatoes, were actually digested and absorbed very quickly (contrary to popular opinion);

- many sugar-containing foods were not the villains responsible for high blood sugar.

Carbohydrate foods that break down quickly during digestion have the highest G.I. values. The blood glucose, or sugar, response is fast and high. In other words, the glucose in the bloodstream increases rapidly. Conversely, carbohydrates that break down slowly, releasing glucose gradually into the bloodstream, have low G.I. values. An analogy might be the popular fable of the tortoise and the hare. The hare, just like high G.I. foods, speeds away full steam ahead but loses the race to the tortoise with his slow and steady pace. Similarly, slow and steady low G.I. foods produce a smooth blood sugar curve without wild fluctuations.

For most people most of the time, the foods with low G.I. values have advantages over those with high G.I. values. The graph below shows the effect of slow and fast carbohydrates on blood sugar levels.

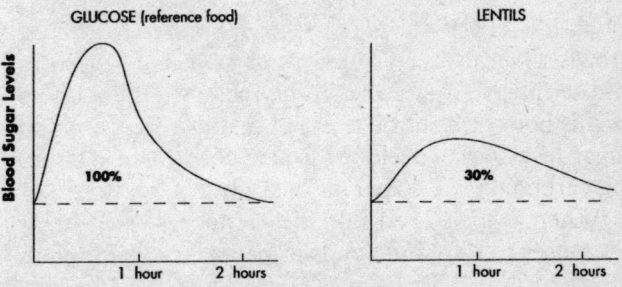

Figure 1. The effect of pure glucose (50 grams) and lentils (50 grams carbohydrate portion) on blood sugar levels.

THE GLYCEMIC INDEX IS:

- a scientifically proven guide to the actual effects of carbohydrate foods on blood sugar levels;
- an easy and effective way to eat a healthy diet and control fluctuations in blood sugar.

THE GLYCEMIC INDEX IS A CLINICALLY PROVEN TOOL IN ITS APPLICATION TO DIABETES, APPETITE CONTROL, AND REDUCING THE RISK OF HEART DISEASE.

Chapter 4

HOW WE MEASURE THE GLYCEMIC INDEX

The substance that produces the greatest rise in blood sugar levels is pure glucose itself. All other foods have less effect when fed in equal amounts of carbohydrate. The glycemic index of pure glucose is set at 100, and every other food is ranked on a scale from 0 to 100 according to its actual effect on blood sugar levels.

We can't predict the glycemic index of a food from its composition or the glycemic index of related foods. To test the glycemic index, we need real people and real foods. There is no easy, inexpensive substitute test. Scientists always follow standardized methods so that results from one group of people can be directly compared with those of another group.

The most important point to note is that all foods

are tested in equivalent carbohydrate amounts. For example, we test 100 grams of bread (about 3½ slices of sandwich bread) because that amount contains 50 grams of carbohydrate. Likewise, 60 grams of jelly beans, containing 50 grams of carbohydrate, are compared with the reference food. We know how much carbohydrate is in a food by consulting food composition tables or the manufacturer's data or by measuring it ourselves in the laboratory.

Scientists use just six steps to determine the glycemic index of a food. Simple as this may sound, it's actually quite a time-consuming process. Here's how it works.

1. An amount of food containing 50 grams of carbohydrate is given to a volunteer to eat. For example, to test boiled spaghetti, the volunteer would be given 200 grams of spaghetti, which supplies 50 grams of carbohydrate (we work this out from food composition tables or by measuring the available carbohydrate). Fifty grams of carbohydrate is equivalent to 3 tablespoons of pure glucose powder.

2. Over the next two hours (or three hours if the volunteer has diabetes), we take a sample of their blood every 15 minutes during the first hour and every 30 minutes thereafter. The blood sugar level of these blood samples is measured in the laboratory and recorded.

3. The blood sugar level is plotted on a graph and the area under the curve is calculated using a computer program (Figure 1).

4. The volunteer's response to spaghetti (or whatever food is being tested) is compared with his or her blood sugar response to 50 grams of pure glucose (the reference food).

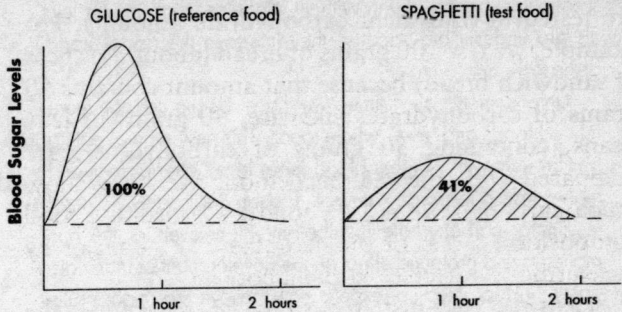

Figure 2. Measuring the glycemic index of a food. The effect of a food on blood sugar levels is calculated using the area under the curve (shaded area). The area under the curve after consumption of the test food is compared with the same area after the reference food (usually 50 grams of pure glucose or a 50 gram carbohydrate portion of white bread).

5. The reference food is tested on two or three separate occasions and an average value is calculated. This is done to reduce the effect of day-to-day variation in blood sugar responses.

6. The average glycemic index found in 8 to 10 people is the glycemic index of that food.

CARBOHYDRATES AND INSULIN

The pancreas is a vital organ near the stomach, and its main job is to produce the hormone insulin. Carbohydrate stimulates the secretion of insulin more than any other component of food. The slow absorption of the carbohydrate in our food means that the pancreas doesn't have to work so hard and needs to produce less insulin. If the pancreas is overstimulated over a long period of time, it may become exhausted and type 2 diabetes can develop in genetically susceptible people. Even without diabetes, high insulin levels are undesirable because they increase the risk of heart disease.

Unfortunately, over time, we have begun to eat more refined foods and fewer whole foods. This new way of eating has brought with it higher blood sugar levels after a meal and higher insulin responses as well. Though our bodies do need insulin for carbohydrate metabolism, high levels of the hormone have a profound effect on the development of many diseases. In fact, medical experts now believe that high insulin levels are one of the key factors responsible for heart disease and hypertension. Insulin influences the way we metabolize foods, determining whether we burn fat or carbohydrate to meet our energy needs and ultimately determining whether we store fat in our bodies.

Chapter 5

WHO BENEFITS FROM LOW G.I. FOODS?

*W*e all do! The slow digestion and gradual rise and fall in blood sugar levels after eating a low G.I. food reduces the secretion of the hormone insulin into the blood. High insulin levels are undesirable because they increase our risk of heart disease, diabetes, and obesity. Reducing this risk is why low G.I. foods benefit everyone—people with and without diabetes. These facts are no exaggeration: They're confirmed by many studies published in prestigious journals around the world.

G.I. VALUE RANGES

Low G.I. foods = below 55
Intermediate G.I. foods = between 55 and 70
High G.I. foods = greater than 70

LOW G.I./HIGH G.I. CHOICES

A food is neither good nor bad based on its glycemic index. For example, if a food is high in fat, it's not a good idea to eat it regularly just because it has a low G.I. value. By the same token, we shouldn't demonize low fat, high G.I. foods like some types of potatoes. The truth is, potatoes make a far better eating option than a food loaded with saturated fat, even if its glycemic index is low.

■

> CONSIDER THE G.I. VALUE OF A FOOD
> IN CONJUNCTION WITH ITS FAT, FIBER, AND
> SALT CONTENT — NOT BY ITSELF.

■

Chapter 6

A HEALTHY DIET FOR CHILDREN

Children are not simply little adults: They're growing all the time—from birth to puberty, for example, your child's skeleton increases sevenfold in size! And at different ages your child has very specific energy and nutrient needs.

Children also have much smaller stomachs than adults, which means that whatever you give them to fill them up must also meet their nutrient needs. For most active children, appetite is the best indicator of how much they need to eat.

Children can also be very fussy eaters. Taste buds undoubtedly dictate some likes and dislikes, but children quickly learn to enjoy or hate foods and can be influenced by how you prepare and present meals, what their friends eat, and what they see advertised on television. Don't despair, though: Healthy children will eat what their bodies need as long as a wide variety of food is available.

A healthy diet for children should:
- maintain good health and growth;
- satisfy their appetite;
- encourage good eating habits;
- promote varied and interesting meals and snacks;
- accommodate a child's usual routines and activities;
- maintain a healthy body weight.

To help your child develop normally, follow these dietary guidelines for childhood and teen nutrition:

- Encourage and support breastfeeding.
- Make sure that your child eats a wide variety of nutritious foods, particularly calcium- and iron-rich foods.
- Steer clear of low fat diets for young children. (For teenagers, diets low in saturated fat, as recommended for adults, are appropriate.)
- Encourage your child to drink plenty of water.
- Make sure that your child gets appropriate food and physical activity.
- Check your child's growth regularly.
- Allow your child to eat only moderate amounts of sugar and foods containing added sugars.
- Choose low salt foods for your child.
- Be sure that your child eats plenty of breads, cereals, vegetables (including legumes), and fruits.

Chapter 7

THE WAY CHILDREN EAT

Most children are natural "grazers"; they usually like to have frequent meals and snacks throughout the day. It's not a good idea to force children to eat everything on their plate if they're already full. Instead, serve them age-appropriate portions of a wide variety of foods. You should also encourage them to eat according to their appetite.

High fiber diets, which are bulky and filling, as well as very low fat diets, generally are unsuitable for young children because it's hard for young ones to eat enough of those foods to meet their energy and nutrient requirements.

Low G.I. foods are suitable for any age and play a large role in children's healthy diets because they:

- include a wide variety of foods,
- allow for individual variation,
- provide long-lasting energy,
- are nutrient dense.

■

REMEMBER!
PARENTS ARE RESPONSIBLE FOR
WHAT IS PROVIDED TO EAT.
CHILDREN ARE RESPONSIBLE FOR HOW MUCH,
AND EVEN WHETHER, THEY EAT.

■

Chapter 8

WHY OUR CHILDREN ARE AT RISK

Today's typical diet tends to be too high in fat and quickly digested carbohydrate foods. Many of the starchy staples, such as potatoes, white bread, breakfast cereals, and rice, that we love to eat also have very high G.I. values. So, too, do most cookies, fat-free muffins and cakes, fat-free frozen desserts, and instant puddings. Unfortunately, these foods may be putting our children and us at risk of obesity, diabetes, and heart disease.

Did you know that about one-third of our school children are overweight? Worse yet, those numbers are rising. Over the past 20 years, the number of overweight children has increased by more than 50%! Why? A combination of too little physical activity and too many "energy dense" convenience foods, as well as supersized meals and snacks, is largely to blame. It's easy to eat too many calories when so many foods are high in hidden fat and quickly digested carbohydrates with little "fill-up" value.

Poor nutrition can affect a child's self-esteem, mental and physical performance, and academic achievement and increase the risk of developing obesity, type 2 diabetes, high blood pressure, and heart disease.

Research has shown that many overweight children also have elevated levels of circulating insulin, which is an early warning sign for type 2 diabetes, a condition doctors previously saw only in adults.

Chapter 9

G.I. VALUES AND CHILDREN'S WEIGHT

We can't overemphasize the importance of helping children learn about good nutrition by providing them with a healthy diet and setting a good example. Offering nutritious and enjoyable food and making mealtimes happy occasions help children develop food preferences that are compatible with good health. It's never too late to start, either. Here's a bonus: By setting a good example, you'll feel more fit and in peak condition, too!

It's easy to incorporate the benefits of low G.I. foods into a healthy diet for children! Eating low G.I. foods is simply part of a sensible, well-balanced and nutritious diet based on scientific evidence regarding carbohydrate metabolism. Evidence has shown that low G.I. foods may help people lose weight, because foods with a low G.I. value also have a higher satiety value (they make you feel fuller after eating) and reduce the food's impact on blood sugar and insulin response. Low G.I foods, combined with a sensible eating schedule and physical activity, will help put a child's weight within the healthy range and keep it there.

■

IF CHILDREN LEARN TO COMBINE
REGULAR PHYSICAL ACTIVITY
WITH HEALTHY LOW G.I. EATING EARLY IN THEIR LIVES,
THEY WILL BE DEVELOPING HEALTHY LIFESTYLE HABITS
THAT MAY CONTINUE INTO ADULTHOOD.

■

A healthy, balanced diet for children today should include a wide variety of foods with the majority of the calories coming from unrefined, fibrous carbohydrates. In the G.I. menus, which start on page 56, we give you plenty of suggestions for breakfast, lunch, dinner, and snacks for children of all ages.

Chapter 10

WHY WE NEED MORE CARBOHYDRATE

Most experts agree that the food we eat for breakfast, lunch, dinner, and in-between snacks should be low in fat and high in carbohydrate. And when it comes to choosing the best fuel for vigorous and extended physical activity—whether it's sports or play—again carbohydrate is the best choice. It's also the only fuel that the brain can use. Studies show that a balanced carbohydrate meal enhances memory and learning; in fact, children's scores on classroom tests are higher if they consume healthy carbohydrates for breakfast.

In addition, carbohydrate and fat have a reciprocal relationship in our diet: if we eat more high carbohydrate foods, they tend to displace the high fat foods from our diet. And when carbohydrate foods (such as a breakfast of Special K™, skim milk, and fruit, instead of a chocolate doughnut) displace saturated and trans fats, they improve the diet's overall nutritional quality. In fact, carbohydrate should be the main source of calories in our food—not fat.

■

**A HEALTHY, BALANCED DIET FOR CHILDREN
CONTAINS A WIDE VARIETY OF FOODS.**

■

Chapter 11

SOURCES OF CARBOHYDRATE

At the beginning of this book we explained that carbohydrate is the fuel our bodies like best. Carbohydrate is important for children because it gives them the energy they need every day to play, study, and take part in sports.

Breads and cereals, vegetables, and fruits are all sources of carbohydrate. Milk products also contain carbohydrate in the form of milk sugar, or lactose, which is the first carbohydrate we consume as babies.

Some foods contain a large amount of carbohydrate (cereals, potatoes, and legumes are good examples), while other foods, such as carrots and broccoli and salad vegetables, are very dilute sources and don't provide nearly enough carbohydrate for our high carbohydrate diet. So, as nutritious as salads can be, they aren't meals on their own; you need to complement them with a carbohydrate food such as whole-grain bread or pasta.

THE BEST HIGH CARBOHYDRATE, LOW FAT CHOICES

Some foods, such as those listed below, are high in carbohydrate and provide very little fat. Your children can eat lots of these foods, as long as you spare the butter, margarine, and oil as you prepare and serve them. We've listed the high G.I. foods in italics.

Cereal grains

These include barley, oats, *popcorn*, rice, rye, wheat, and anything made from them, such as bread, breakfast cereals, flour, noodles, pasta, polenta, and ravioli.
Servings per day: 4 or more

Fruits

These include apples, apricots, *bananas*, cherries, grapes, kiwifruit, mangoes, melons, oranges, peaches, pears, *pineapples*, and plums. Serve them whole or as juices and smoothies.
Servings per day: 3 or more

Vegetables

Vegetables provide valuable amounts of vitamins, minerals, and fiber. You can eat most vegetables without thinking about their G.I. value because they're very low in carbohydrate. The higher carbohydrate vegetables for filling, satisfying meals include potatoes, corn, peas, and sweet potatoes. Of these, corn and sweet potatoes are the lower G.I. choices.
Servings per day: 4 or more

Beans, peas, and legumes

Baked beans, chickpeas, kidney beans, lentils, and split peas are protein-rich, high carbohydrate, low G.I. choices. Serve them as light meals, soups, and salads.

Servings per day: 1

Milk and milk products

Milk and dairy foods such as custard, pudding, ice cream, and yogurt are excellent sources of carbohydrate and calcium. If they want, teenagers can use low fat milk products to minimize their fat intake.

Servings per day: 3 to 4

Chapter 12

LOW G.I. DIETS FOR CHILDREN

It's easy to incorporate low G.I. foods into a child's diet and rewarding to watch him or her reap the benefits. It usually just means making a few substitutions, such as those shown on page 29. Ideally, you should aim to swap at least half of the high G.I. foods that you give children for low G.I. choices. For example, you could change the type of bread or breakfast cereal and serve pasta or legumes more often. And don't forget milk and dairy foods.

Remember that it isn't necessary to serve children only low G.I. foods. On the contrary, meals usually consist of a variety of foods, and eating a low G.I. food with a high G.I. food produces an intermediate G.I. meal. Here are three ways to make serving low G.I. foods easier:

- Become familiar with the different types of low G.I. choices available.
- Have low G.I. foods available in the pantry and refrigerator.
- Experiment with new foods and recipes.

■

TRY TO INCLUDE AT LEAST ONE LOW G.I. FOOD PER MEAL PER DAY.

■

SUBSTITUTING LOW G.I. FOR HIGH G.I. FOODS

High G.I. Food	Low G.I. Alternative
Bread, whole-wheat or white	Bread containing lots of "grainy bits" that is dense, heavy, and usually dark, such as 100% stone-ground whole-wheat, wholegrain pumpernickel, and sourdough rye
Most processed breakfast cereals, such as cornflakes, Rice/Corn Chex, Rice Krispies, Crispix, and Shredded Wheat	Unrefined cereals such as rolled oats or muesli or a low G.I. processed cereal such as All Bran and Special K™
Crackers, such as saltines, Ritz, Wheatables, and rice cakes; cookies such as sugar wafers, Snackwells and Oreos	Crackers such as WASA, Ry Krisp, Kavli, and Ryvita; cookies such as graham crackers, oatmeal, Social Tea and Lorna Doones
Most cakes and muffins	Muffins made with fruit, oats, and 100% whole-wheat flour
Tropical fruits such as bananas, pineapple, watermelon, and raisins	Temperate-climate fruits such as apples, pears, peaches, nectarines, all berries, and grapes

THE GLUCOSE REVOLUTION POCKET GUIDE

High G.I. Food	Low G.I. Alternative
White potatoes, baked or mashed	Baby new potatoes, sweet potatoes, corn, pasta, and legumes
Short-grain or "sticky" rice grain, basmati, or brown rice	Uncle Ben's Converted rice or any other long-

Chapter 13

FOOD BASICS

*N*ow that you know about the glycemic index, here's how some popular foods fit into a low G.I. lifestyle.

CEREALS AND GRAINS

Today, cereal and grains are major sources of energy and protein for people all over the world, but they weren't part of the diet that humankind evolved on millions of years ago. As human populations grew, resources of mammals, fish, and birds became depleted. It's been only over the last 10,000 years that we've begun to rely more on cereals for food—with consequent developments in processing.

Unprocessed cereals and grains are naturally slowly digested foods. In early times, they were roughly ground between stones, which broke the outer seed husk but left much of the grain intact and produced a coarse meal. Today, cereal processing includes milling the grain into a fine flour, then popping, toasting, flaking, and extrusion cooking to make cakes, breads, cookies, snack products, and breakfast cereals.

One of the nutritional implications of this dietary change has been an increase in the G.I. value, because modern processing methods transform the low G.I. carbohydrate of cereal grains into high G.I. foods. In other words, because of the processing, or refinement, of whole grains, our bodies have much less work to do to digest them into blood sugar (glucose) and dump them into the bloodstream.

To eat a low G.I. diet, choose less-processed cereal products and whole-grain cereals. Hint: The higher the fiber content, the more intact the grains are. Aim for 5 grams of fiber or more per serving.

PASTA

Most children love pasta. And not only is it good to eat, it's good to eat it often, because whether you choose penne or spaghetti or fettuccine, you are choosing one of nature's naturally low G.I. foods.

Most pasta is made from semolina (finely cracked wheat), which is milled from very hard wheat with a high protein content. A stiff dough, made by mixing the semolina with water, is forced through a die and dried. There is very little disruption of the starch granule during this process, and the strong protein-starch interactions inhibit starch gelatinization. The dense consistency also makes the pasta resistant to disruption in the small intestine and contributes to the final low glycemic index—even pasta made from fine flour (instead of semolina) has a relatively low glycemic index. There's some evidence that thicker pasta has a lower glycemic index than thin types because of its dense consistency and perhaps because it cooks more slowly. (It's also less likely to be overcooked.) The addition of egg to fresh pasta lowers the G.I. value by increasing the protein content: Higher protein levels slow stomach emptying, because only about 60% of the protein gets broken down; the rest goes into storage as fat.

Italians eat their pasta al dente, which literally means "to the tooth." It must be slightly firm and offer some resistance when you're chewing it. Not only does al dente pasta taste better than soft, soggy pasta, but it also has a lower G.I. value, because overcooking pasta increases starch gelatinization, or swelling, and boosts its glycemic index.

■

OUR BOOKS *THE GLUCOSE REVOLUTION* AND *THE GLUCOSE REVOLUTION LIFE PLAN* HAVE MANY RECIPES THAT YOUR WHOLE FAMILY WILL ENJOY.

■

RICE

Rice is an ideal accompaniment to spicy foods. Milling rice removes the bran and germ, which results in a considerable nutrient loss. Brown rice is a better source of B vitamins, minerals, and fiber; be sure to vary your family's diet to include both brown and white rice. And look for other lower G.I. rices, including Uncle Ben's Converted and basmati rice, in your supermarket.

BREAD

One of the most important changes you can make to lower the G.I. value of your children's diet is to choose a low G.I. bread when making toast, sandwiches, or snacks.

Eat dense breads that contain a lot of whole grains: If the fibrous seed coat of cereal grains is intact, it acts as a physical barrier to slow down starch digestion. Pumpernickel is a true whole-grain bread—it's made from whole rye grains.

Other low G.I. breads include sourdough and stone-ground flour breads, types that don't contain any enriched wheat flour. The acids in sourdough breads may reduce the glycemic index, the acids that result from fermentation of the starch and sugars are believed to lower G.I. values by slowing down stomach emptying. To add more bread to your child's meals, read our sandwich suggestions for snacks and school lunches on pages 62 and 67.

If you're making your own bread, you can add your own G.I.-lowering ingredients, such as linseed, flaxseed, rolled oats, cornmeal, oat bran, barley meal, cracked wheat, and wheat berries.

VEGETABLES

You and your children can eat most vegetables without thinking about their glycemic index. Most are so low in carbohydrate that they have no measurable effect on our blood sugar levels, but they still provide valuable amounts of fiber, vitamins, and minerals. Higher carbohydrate vegetables include potatoes, sweet potatoes, corn, and peas. Among these, corn and sweet potatoes are the lower G.I. choices. Pumpkin, carrots, peas, and beets contain some carbohydrate, but a half-cup serving contains so little that these foods don't raise blood sugar levels significantly.

Salad vegetables such as tomatoes, lettuce, cucumbers, peppers, and onions also have so little carbohydrate that it's impossible to test their glycemic index values. In generous serving sizes, they won't have any effect on blood sugar. Think of them as "free" foods that are full of healthful micronutrients. Eat and enjoy!

FRUIT

Not only does fruit make an ideal snack, you can transform it into a tasty sweet dessert quickly and easily. Fruit contains carbohydrate, fiber, vitamins (such as vitamin C and beta-carotene), and minerals. Most fresh fruit contains vitamin C, so all of us—not just our children—should eat it every day, preferably whole, rather than as juice.

Most fruits have low G.I. values thanks to the low glycemic index of fructose, a major sugar in fruit. The presence of viscous fiber, such as pectin and acids (which may slow down stomach emptying), also help keep the glycemic index low.

- Fruits with the lowest G.I. values tend to be those grown in temperate climates, such as apples, pears, citrus, peaches, plums, cherries and all berries.

- The more acidic the fruit, the lower its glycemic index; for example, grapefruit's glycemic index is 25.
- Tropical fruits, such as melons, pineapples, and bananas, have intermediate G.I. values.

DAIRY FOODS

You should encourage your children to eat dairy foods throughout their childhood and beyond. Not only are dairy foods an important source of calcium, but they also have low G.I. values. Dairy foods also provide energy, protein, carbohydrate, vitamin B_2, and important fat-soluble vitamins such as vitamins A and D.

If for some reason your child is allergic to cow's milk, try a lactose-free milk or suitable calcium-fortified soy substitute (approximately 180 mg of calcium per 4 ounces). The soy drinks that we have tested have low G.I. values similar to those of cow's milk. The good news is that most children will outgrow a cow's milk allergy by five years of age.

Calcium helps build and maintain strong bones and teeth and has other important nerve and muscle functions. Milk, yogurt, ice cream, pudding, and custard are all excellent low G.I. sources of calcium. Cheese, although a good source of calcium, is considered a source of protein rather than carbohydrate and contains no lactose.

For answers to some of your most-asked dairy questions, turn to pages 85.

BREAST IS STILL BEST

Experts highly recommend breast milk for all infants—it's convenient and nutritionally complete and has immunological properties that provide greater resistance to infections and diseases. It also enhances the bonding between mother and infant. Feeding your infant when he or she is hungry will provide all the energy and nutrient requirements needed for normal growth and development.

But how do you know if your child is getting enough? Be reassured: Your child is getting enough milk if he or she is gaining weight and producing a satisfactory number of wet diapers.

If breastfeeding is not an option, choose a suitable fortified infant formula and offer your baby a bottle every three or four hours.

Breast milk or infant formula should be your baby's main drink until he or she is about 12 months old. From about 7 months you can introduce whole cow's milk (pasteurized and homogenized) in small quantities as custard, yogurt, or on cereal. After 12 months, when your child is eating a varied diet, you can offer whole cow's milk as the main drink.

MEAT AND MEAT ALTERNATIVES

Proteins are the body's building blocks, so we need to eat a variety of protein foods from animal or plant sources to create, maintain, and renew our body cells. Children and teenagers, because they are growing, need more protein in relation to their body weight than adults do; they are building new body cells.

- Red meat, chicken, pork, and fish are important sources of protein and micronutrients such as iron. They don't contain carbohydrate, so they don't have a G.I. value. Choose lean meats where possible; there are now many trim cuts available. Serve *infrequently* such fatty processed meats as sausage, frankfurters, chicken nuggets and salami.
- Include fish in the family meals at least once a week, especially tuna or salmon, which are high in heart-healthy omega-3 essential fatty acids.
- Legumes such as split peas, baked beans, and lentils provide protein, vitamin B, and iron, as does meat, but legumes are also excellent low G.I. sources of carbohydrate. Try to incorporate them in family meals at least once a week.

NATURAL PEANUT BUTTER

Natural peanut butter is a high protein, nutrient-dense food. It contains fiber, iron, and heart-healthy monounsaturated fat. Peanut butter and all-fruit jelly on whole-grain bread is a great breakfast, lunch, or snack that requires little time or skill to prepare! And just for variety, you can try other nut butters, such as cashew, almond, and soy.

FATS AND OILS

Although we need a moderate amount of fat as an energy source, such as fat from essential fatty acids and fat-soluble vitamins, we rarely have to go out of our way to consume enough of them.

There are different types of fat in foods, and saturated fats and trans-fatty acids are the most heart *un*healthy. Solid at room temperature, saturated fat comes in the form of fatty marbling in meat, the cream in milk and other high fat dairy products, and some of the tropical oils, such as palm oil, widely used as shortening for frying and for making cakes, pies, cookies, and crackers. Many studies from all around the world clearly have shown that saturated fat increases our risk of coronary heart disease.

Trans-fatty acids are produced during the manufacture of margarines and behave like saturated fat in the products, increasing their firmness, as well as in our bodies, increasing the risk of heart attack. Foods high in trans fats include fried fast foods, some margarines, crackers, cookies, and snack cakes.

Nuts, lean meats, avocadoes, and foods made with polyunsaturated or monounsaturated fats and oils, on the other hand, all contain heart-healthy fats. Try to plan meals and snacks with these foods in mind.

DON'T THROW THE BABY OUT WITH THE BATH WATER! SOME FATS ARE ESSENTIAL FOR HEALTHY BODIES. ONLY SATURATED FATS AND TRANS FATS SHOULD BE KEPT TO A MINIMUM.

Young children (under five) need fat for energy and shouldn't be put on a low fat diet unless they are under strict medical supervision. You can offer reduced fat products to older children with larger appetites.

Chapter 14

SUGAR 101

Children naturally enjoy sweet foods. Sweetness is not a learned taste; in fact, it could be said that we're all born with a sweet tooth. Not only is our first food, breast milk, sweet, but also infants smile when offered a sweet solution, as they reject sour and bitter tastes.

Did you know that a balanced diet should include some fat and sugar? Studies over the past decade have found that high sugar diets are no less nutritious than diets containing lower amounts of sugar: When we restrict sugar, we frequently eat more fat, and the most popular fatty foods are poor sources of nutrients. In some cases, high sugar diets may have higher micronutrient contents, because sugar is often used to sweeten some very nutritious foods, such as yogurts, breakfast cereals, and milk.

Today, glycemic index researchers have tested hundreds of real foods on real people, and the results are surprising: Sugar is not the dietary demon that it was once made out to be. Many Americans, though, eat far too much of it. Sixteen percent of our average daily caloric intake comes from sweeteners (health experts recommend 6 to 10%). That's why each of us needs to look at our own diet and adjust our sugar intake accordingly. You and your children can enjoy sugar and foods containing sugar *in moderation* as part of a balanced low G.I. diet.

WHAT EXACTLY IS "MODERATE INTAKE"?

A moderate intake of refined sugar for a child is between 7 to 12 teaspoonfuls a day. Keep in mind that we're talking about the sugar found in foods, such as all non-diet soft drinks, breakfast cereals, candy, ice cream, cookies, jelly, and syrups. Adding a *small* amount of sugar to a well-balanced, low G.I. diet can make foods taste better and make them more acceptable to children without compromising their nutritional intake or the benefits of the low G.I. foods.

SUGARY FOODS AND DENTAL CAVITIES

Most of what we know about the relationship between sugar and dental cavities came from the pre-fluoride era of long ago. Children who have been exposed to fluoride all their lives have little or no dental decay despite a high sugar intake. Obviously, regular toothbrushing plays a more important role in the prevention of tooth decay.

A MODERATE-SUGAR MENU

This child's menu provides 46 grams (about 12 teaspoons) of refined sugars and approximately 1500 calories with 25% of energy from fat and 56% of energy from carbohydrate.

Breakfast
¾ cup Special K with 4 oz. 1% milk
½ cup strawberries
4 oz. apple juice

Snack options
4 oz. natural applesauce (snack pack)

Lunch
Grilled cheese on 100% whole-wheat bread
6–8 baby carrots
Cinnamon Teddy Grahams (snack pack)
4 oz. low fat chocolate milk

Snack
Quaker Chewy low fat granola bar
4 oz. 1% milk

Dinner
3 oz. meatloaf
½ cup green beans with 1 pat butter
½ cup candied yams
¾ cup melon balls
4 oz. 1% milk

Snack
 ½ cup chocolate or butterscotch pudding (snack pack)

THE ROLE OF ARTIFICIALLY SWEETENED PRODUCTS IN CHILDREN'S DIETS

While artificially sweetened products may sometimes be appropriate for overweight children, they aren't necessary for the average child. Many of these products, such as diet sodas and sugar-free candies and sweets, are simply flavored fillers and provide few, if any, nutrients. It is nutritionally unwise to allow children to fill up on calorie-free, nutrient-*free* foods—we should serve them nutrient-*packed* foods instead.

SUGAR AND BEHAVIOR

Although some people believe that sugar causes attention deficit disorder or hyperactivity in children, results from many published studies have failed to provide any scientifically proven support for this claim. In studies in which the investigator, the child, and the parent were unaware of the test food or capsule, refined sugar had no effect on cognitive performance, nor did it cause or worsen hyperactivity.

It is possible that a *very* small number of children may respond adversely to fluctuations in blood sugar levels caused by sugar. But if this is the case, any high G.I. carbohydrate, including bread and potatoes, will also be incriminated.

On the whole, there is more evidence that sugar might actually have a calming effect if it has any effect at all. Glucose or sugar can reduce the distress associated with painful medical procedures in infants. In one study, infants subjected to heel pricks cried less and had lower heart rates when they were given a sugar solution immediately prior to the procedure, compared with children who were given just water.

Chapter 15

ACTIVITY AND SPORTS

*E*xercise and physical activity are important to help your child stay fit and maintain a healthy body weight. Encourage your child to be active every day, whether it's through playing a sport, enjoying a hobby, playing outdoors, or walking the dog. As a family, you can enjoy walking, swimming, bicycle riding in the park, or playing catch with a football or basketball.

Toddlers rarely need encouragement to be active; they're usually on the go all day long. School children, on the other hand, often sit at their desks for long periods of time. Physical education classes and sports are important in that they not only help your child develop physical skills, but also help build confidence and self-esteem.

Too often teenagers need (or choose) to remain inactive as they do homework, watch television, or work part-time. They often opt out of sports, which can make it difficult for them to begin playing one later on. That's why you need to encourage your teenagers to be active. Let them know that exercise—not dieting—is the best way to stay in good shape.

■

TURN OFF THE TELEVISION AND THE COMPUTER
AND ENCOURAGE YOUR KIDS TO BE ACTIVE
FOR AT LEAST AN HOUR A DAY.

■

FOUR TIPS TO KEEP YOUR CHILDREN ACTIVE

1. Encourage children to participate in physical activities in their spare time. It's better that they be out riding a bike, in-line skating, or swimming than watching television or playing computer games.
2. Encourage interests that work around their usual busy schedule, such as an activity that's on the way to or from school.
3. Help them learn the basic skills of several activities to give them the confidence and ability to participate.
4. Set a good example and join in the fun!

Regular daily activity
- gives children a more positive attitude toward healthy lifestyle habits;
- stimulates the basal metabolic rate (BMR), the rate at which we produce and use energy while we're at total rest (the BMR primarily determines how many calories we will burn each day);
- increases energy output;
- allows children more flexibility in their diet;
- maintains a healthy body weight.

Chapter 16

EAT TO COMPETE

When it comes to sports performance, eating well can be just as important as training and practice sessions! A diet rich in carbohydrate works best for active people because carbohydrate is the best fuel for working muscles. Keep these tips in mind as you plan meals and snacks for active kids:

- Make healthy food choices a part of sporting events by taking something with you. Great snacks to pack include fresh fruit, sandwiches, muffins, low fat granola bars, yogurt, milk drinks, fruit juices, dried fruit and nuts, hot soup, and crusty rolls and toasted sandwiches.
- Prepare for the inevitable hunger pangs when

children come home from a sporting event by having quick high carbohydrate meals on hand. Some good examples include pasta with tomato sauce and grated cheese, stir-fried vegetables and noodles, peanut butter and all-fruit jelly sandwiches, and canned soups such as lentil, split pea, or minestrone.
- Encourage your child to drink lots of fluids during and after exercise. Remember: Thirst doesn't adequately indicate that our bodies need water. In most cases water is sufficient, but flavored water or seltzer may encourage kids to drink more liquid. (Commercial sports drinks also have this advantage.) Juicy fruits like sliced melon or grapes are also great for providing fluid and carbohydrate simultaneously. Instead of routinely offering orange sections, serve your kids fresh strawberries.

IF YOUR CHILD IS INVOLVED IN ENDURANCE SPORTS

If your child participates in sports, you can use both low G.I. and high G.I. foods to enhance his or her performance. Here's how.

Pre-event eating
Researchers at the University of Sydney found that a low G.I. pre-event meal can delay fatigue by delivering carbohydrate to muscles late in exercise. Because they are slowly digested, low G.I. foods eaten at least one hour before endurance events can act as a slow-release fuel supply, providing glucose at the time when glycogen stores are running low. (Glycogen is a limited amount of energy stored as starch in the mus-

cles for quick conversion into sugar for energy.)

It's important to serve the same foods during the training period as you plan to use on the actual day of competition so you know in advance that the foods deliver the energy needed and that your child can tolerate them.

Good pre-event foods
- Yogurt
- Sandwich made with low G.I. bread
- Low G.I. breakfast cereals
- Low G.I. fruit
- Fruit smoothies
- Pasta

Post-event eating

Right after an athletic event, high G.I. foods are the best choice. Since they are quickly absorbed, they're ideal for replenishing depleted glycogen stores after exercise. High G.I. foods are particularly important when your child has two or more strenuous training sessions every day. When more exercise is scheduled for later in the day, make sure your child eats or drinks carbohydrate within 30 minutes of the first session.

Good choices after competition
- Sports drinks
- Rice cakes with jam
- White bread and honey
- Cookies and fruit juice
- Cornflakes or Rice Krispies

Chapter 17

TIPS FOR LOWER G.I. MEALS

*P*lanning low G.I. meals means using a wide variety of fresh, tasty foods. And it's easy to modify most of your favorite recipes to lower their glycemic index: Changing just one ingredient in a recipe can be enough to lower the G.I. value of the whole meal! Here are some examples to give you ideas:

- Make a minestrone by adding lentils, barley, split peas, beans, or pasta to soup.
- In casseroles, substitute red or pink kidney beans, cannellini beans, or chickpeas for a portion of the meat. It boosts the fiber and lowers the fat, too.

- For meatballs or meatloaf, add mashed cooked or canned beans or rolled oats to the minced meat.

Alternatively, serve the meal with low G.I. accompaniments such as a low G.I. bread, al dente pasta, low G.I. rice, sweet potatoes, or corn, or serve a dessert made with apples, pears, peaches, or plums.

Chapter 18

THE FOOD PYRAMID FOR CHILDREN

School-age children have changing energy needs due to their growth rate, body size and physical activity level. All children need at least the minimum number of servings from each of the five food groups every day. Older, larger, and more active children will require the maximum number of servings, which will give their bodies the 1800 to 2200 calories they require for proper growth and good health.

THE FOOD PYRAMID FOR CHILDREN

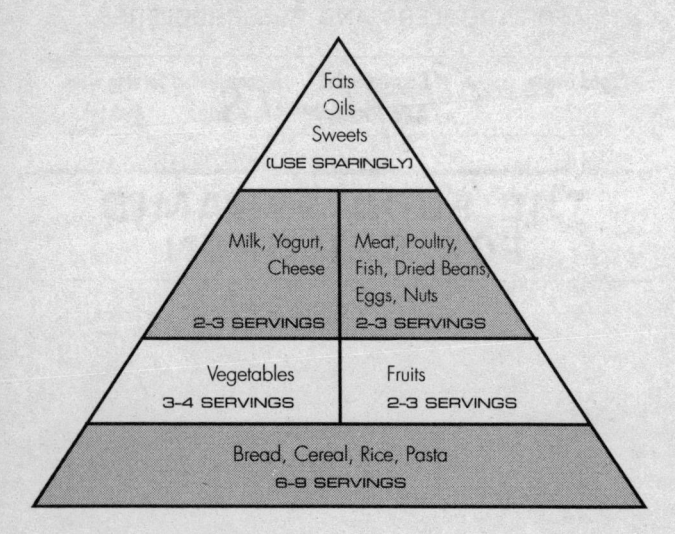

- Fats, Oils, Sweets (USE SPARINGLY)
- Milk, Yogurt, Cheese — 2-3 SERVINGS
- Meat, Poultry, Fish, Dried Beans, Eggs, Nuts — 2-3 SERVINGS
- Vegetables — 3-4 SERVINGS
- Fruits — 2-3 SERVINGS
- Bread, Cereal, Rice, Pasta — 6-9 SERVINGS

IS YOUR CHILD GETTING ENOUGH WATER?

Water Requirements	Oz. Per Lb./Day
0–3 mos.	1.2–2.5
4–6 mos.	2.0–2.3
7–12 mos.	1.8–2.0
1 year	1.8–2.0
2 years	1.7–1.9
6 years	1.4–1.3

RECOMMENDED DAILY QUANTITIES OF FOOD FOR TODDLERS AND PRESCHOOLERS

Food Group	Recommended Daily Servings	Recommended Serving Sizes 1–3 yrs.	4–5 yrs.
Bread (low G.I.)		¼–½ slice	1 slice
Crackers (low G.I.)	≥6	2–3	4–6
Dry cereal (low G.I.)		¼–⅓ cup	½ cup
Cooked cereal, rice, pasta (low G.I.)		¼–⅓ cup	⅓ cup
Fruits and vegetables (low G.I.)	≥5	¼–⅓ cup ½ piece	¼–½ cup ½ piece
Milk, yogurt	≥3	½ cup (4 oz.)	¾ cup (6 oz.)
Lean meat, fish, poultry		1–2 oz.	2–3 oz.
Cheese	≥2	½ oz.	¾ oz.
Eggs		1	1
Dried peas, beans	1–3 tbsp.	1–3 tbsp.	
Margarine, butter, oil	3–4	1 tsp.	1 tsp.

SOURCE: *Manual for Clinical Dietetics*, 5th Ed. (Chicago: The American Dietetic Association, 1996).

Chapter 19

A WEEK OF LOW G.I. MENUS

This week of menus gives you some ideas for including low G.I. foods in your family fare. Be sure to include low G.I. beverages, too.

Note: For the menus below, follow the portion sizes listed in "Recommended Daily Quantities of Food for Toddlers and Preschoolers" on page 55 and "The Food Pyramid for Children" on page 54.

THE GLYCEMIC INDEX AND HEALTHY KIDS

■ MONDAY

Breakfast
   Strawberry-banana smoothie with vanilla yogurt and honey

Snack
   Graham crackers

Lunch
   Ham sandwich with lettuce and tomatoes
   Small apple and mini yogurt

Snack
   Orange quarters

Dinner
   Barbecued chicken with corn on the cob and salad
   Low fat chocolate pudding
   Pear halves

■ TUESDAY

Breakfast
   Sourdough English muffin with spreadable cheese
   Bowl of fruit salad with low fat or light yogurt

Snack
   Low fat granola bar

Lunch
Turkey and tomato sandwich on low G.I. bread, spread with light mayonnaise
Sliced fresh fruit

Snack
Low fat chocolate milk

Dinner
Oven-fried fish sticks (Choose products cooked in canola oil.)
Steamed broccoli
Peaches

■

WEDNESDAY

Breakfast
Low G.I. toast with peanut butter and all-fruit jelly

Snack
Low fat or light yogurt

Lunch
Melted cheese sandwich made with low G.I. bread

Snack
Grapes

Dinner
Chunky chicken-vegetable noodle soup
Whole-grain roll spread with tub margarine
Baked apple

THURSDAY

Breakfast
  Special K™ with skim or low fat milk
  Strawberries or peaches

Snack
  Natural applesauce (snack pack)

Lunch
  Tuna salad sandwich made with low G.I. bread
  Grapes

Snack
  Low fat or light fruit yogurt and sliced fresh fruit

Dinner
  Hamburger on 100% whole wheat bun
  Baked beans
  Large tossed salad
  Low fat chocolate milk

FRIDAY

Breakfast
  Scrambled egg
  Whole-grain toast spread with tub margarine

Snack
  Slice of cheese and whole-wheat crackers

Lunch
Peanut butter and all-fruit jelly on low G.I. bread
Snack pack of peaches

Snack
Fruit yogurt
Chocolate chip cookies

Dinner
Lasagna
Tossed salad
Fresh strawberries with a scoop of low fat ice cream

■

SATURDAY

Breakfast
Sourdough French toast with maple syrup
Sliced fruit

Snack
Oatmeal cookies
Skim or low fat milk

Lunch
Pita pizza
Tossed green salad
Milk

Snack
Baby carrots

THE GLYCEMIC INDEX AND HEALTHY KIDS

Dinner
    Vegetable and noodle stir-fry
    Low fat ice cream with sliced banana, nuts, and chocolate syrup

■

SUNDAY

Breakfast
    Buckwheat pancakes with maple syrup and sliced fruit
    Hot chocolate

Snack
    Piece of fresh fruit

Lunch
    Spaghetti with pasta sauce and cheese
    Bowl of small chunks of fresh fruit offered with toothpicks and yogurt to dip

Snack
    Cheese and fruit plate with water crackers

Dinner
    Lean roast beef with mashed sweet potatoes and green beans
    Apple crisp

Chapter 20

SNACKS AND LIGHT MEALS

*L*ow G.I. foods, as part of your children's meals and snacks, provide the long-term energy your young ones need to make it through a busy day. Here are some tasty choices to consider.

Dairy-based snacks
Milk and no-sugar-added hot chocolate
Fruit smoothies (strawberry, apricot, peach)
Ice cream in a cone
Frozen yogurt in a cone
Yogurt (plain or flavored) mixed with fruit, nuts, Grape-Nuts, or granola

THE GLYCEMIC INDEX AND HEALTHY KIDS 63

Fruit- or vegetable-based snacks
Cheese wedges and dried fruit combo (apples, grapes, apricots, and pears)
Fruit kebabs (fresh fruit wedges on a skewer)
Dips served with pieces of fruit (peach, pear, apple, grapes, orange) or vegetables
Steamed new potatoes served with melted cheese and broccoli
Corn on the cob

Bread- and cereal-based snacks
Cheese or dips with whole-grain crackers or toast
Spaghetti with tomato sauce
Macaroni and cheese
Peanut butter and all-fruit jelly on graham crackers or Ry Krisp
French toast
Leftovers: pizza, rice, noodles
Pancakes or waffles
Muffins or raisin bread with margarine
Pita bread with hummus
Corn chips with melted cheese or salsa (nachos)
Mini pizzas made with pocketless pita or low G.I. English muffins
½ bagel (pumpernickel or sourdough) with ham, cheese, or peanut butter
Vegetable soup with a crusty whole-grain roll
Breakfast cereals (preferably low G.I. varieties) with milk
Grilled or fresh sandwiches (see page 68 for sandwich ideas)

Chapter 21

BREAKFAST BASICS

Breakfast is the meal that starts the day. It's a great opportunity to optimize your use of low G.I. foods because so many breakfast foods—breads, cereals, fresh fruits, and dairy foods—are excellent low G.I. food sources. Studies have shown that children who eat a nutritious breakfast will perform better, both physically and mentally, than their hungry peers. A wholesome, nutritious low G.I. breakfast ensures optimal performance until the scheduled morning snack. Just make sure that your kids have enough time to enjoy their breakfast without feeling rushed.

Though breakfast is important, many children don't have large appetites at breakfast time. For small appetites, fruit smoothies and hot chocolate are good starters that will sustain energy levels throughout the morning. Here are some other ideas.

1. **Start with some fruit.**
   Fruit contributes fiber and vitamin C, which helps your body absorb iron.
2. **Try some breakfast cereal.**
   Cereals are important as a source of fiber, vitamin B, and iron. When choosing processed breakfast cereals, look for those with a high fiber content (five or more grams per serving). The top four low G.I. cereals for children are old-fashioned oats, granola, Life, and Special K™.
3. **Add milk or yogurt.**
   Fat-free or low fat milk can make a valuable contribution to your child's daily calcium intake when you include it at breakfast. Both kinds have low G.I. values, and low fat milk varieties have just as much calcium as whole milk, if not more.
4. **Serve some bread or toast.**
   The lowest G.I. breads are whole-grain pumpernickel (G.I. 51); sourdough (G.I. 52); 100% stone-ground whole wheat (G.I. 53); Arnold's sourdough rye (G.I. 57); and whole-wheat pita (G.I. 57).

Breakfast suggestions
Cereal with milk and fruit
Toasted whole-grain sandwich or toast with peanut butter and all-fruit jelly, cheese, or ham and egg
Bagel or muffin with all-fruit jelly
French toast with fresh fruit

Fruit smoothies
Old-fashioned oats with peaches or natural applesauce
Grilled tomato, ham, and cheese on toast or muffins
Poached egg on toast
Yogurt and fresh fruit
Multigrain waffle and ham
Buckwheat pancakes and stewed peaches or fresh berries

Chapter 22

SCHOOL LUNCH!

Busy school days mean that children need foods that keep them going all day long—to help prevent fatigue, maintain their concentration levels during class, and keep them vital and healthy. Once they're at school, children can't graze throughout the day, so the foods they eat for breakfast, recess, lunch, and after-school snacks must provide them with the long-lasting energy and good nutrition that they require.

Be sure to pack enough food items to cover morning recess, lunch, and possibly beyond, to allow for a fluctuating appetite, since a hungry child won't be able to function at his mental or physical peak. Children who don't eat enough at meal- or snacktime often crave junk foods or binge later. Classic examples are the breakfast skippers who eat large, high calorie mid-morning snacks and the small-school-lunch eaters who come home ravenously hungry and raid the fridge, leaving no appetite for dinner.

FOUR TIPS FOR HEALTHY LUNCHES

1. Use different types of bread for variety: wholegrain, white, sourdough, rye, raisin, pita, herb bread, muffins, semolina rolls and tortilla wraps. Try to select a low G.I. variety whenever you can.

2. Cook toasted sandwiches such as grilled cheese the night before; children can eat them cool for lunch the next day for something a little different.

3. Don't worry if children select the same foods for their lunch box every day as long as their food choices are mainly healthy. They'll let you know when they're bored and ready for more variety.

4. Make sure that you pack enough food each day to meet your child's needs for lunch, snacks, sports, and unexpected extras. Remember: Low G.I. food choices are more sustaining and will help provide the energy levels necessary to last throughout the day—in the classroom, on the playground, and on the sports field.

Sandwich Suggestions
Tuna salad with lettuce and tomato
Egg salad with lettuce and tomato
Crabmeat salad or salmon cakes
Cheese with lettuce and tomato
Cheese with marinated or roasted vegetables
Fried egg

Hummus
Peanut butter and all-fruit jelly
Cold cuts (turkey, ham, roast beef) with pickles or salad/coleslaw and with mayonnaise
Grilled sausages or low fat hot dogs
Grilled chicken breast or chicken salad
Cream cheese and all-fruit jelly
Crispy bacon, tomato, and lettuce
Grated carrot and apple with cream cheese
Ham and cheese on low G.I. English muffin
Avocado, chicken, and ricotta roll-ups (ricotta, avocado, lemon juice, alfalfa sprouts, grated carrot, and chicken rolled in pita bread)
Crunchy chicken (chicken, diced celery, diced apple, grated carrot, and cream cheese)
Grilled ham and/or cheese
Wraps with sliced ham, chicken, turkey, roast beef, cheese, and vegetables

THE LUNCH BOX

When it comes to packing your child's lunch, let your imagination be your guide! Try these ideas for starters.

BREAD	+FRUIT	+DAIRY	+DRINK	+SNACKS
Be adventurous with bread choices. Include different bread varieties, rolls, crispbreads,	Include fresh fruit in season — whole, chopped, diced, or sliced. Also serve fruit packs (in natural	Include milk (plain or flavored), yogurt (natural, vanilla, or flavored), and	You can vary drink choices daily; they can include milk, water, flavored seltzers, or	Check the list on page 62 for a wide variety of nourishing, healthy snacks to include in your child's

BREAD	+FRUIT	+DAIRY	+DRINK	+SNACKS
crackers, and muffins.	juice) and dried fruits.	cheese.	fruit juices on occasion. Freeze drinks in summer and store in your child's lunch box to keep the contents cool.	lunch box.

Chapter 23

THE LATE-MORNING BLAHS

Many very young schoolchildren feel a distinct energy deficit right before late-morning recess. Why? Because the gap between breakfast and recess may be too long and concentration levels may wane, particularly in children who have eaten poorly at breakfast—or worse—eaten no breakfast at all. Check the low G.I. breakfast list on page 65 for ideas on making this important meal more appealing.

If your child has never been one to eat much at breakfast, he or she may benefit from having an additional low G.I. snack on the way to school to help provide that lasting energy. You might like to try dried fruit, flavored milk, a small container of yogurt, or whole-grain crackers with cheese spread or peanut butter and all-fruit jelly.

The opposite timing problem may exist for some students; that is, their lunch period is scheduled very early (for example, before 11:00 A.M.). This is more likely to occur in the upper grades and in high school. To best manage this situation, you should give your child the choice of either a large breakfast, smaller lunch, and then a substantial after-school snack to last him or her until dinnertime or a small but still low G.I., breakfast, normal-size lunch, small snack, and then dinner. Discuss the options with your child and try his or her preference first.

Chapter 24

WHAT'S FOR DINNER?

*P*lanning a low G.I. meal is as easy as 1-2-3 (almost!). Here's all you need to do to get started.

1. **First choose the carbohydrate.**

   As you know, your choices include sweet potatoes, rice (Uncle Ben's Converted or brown), any type of pasta, grains such as cracked wheat or barley, chickpeas, lentils, and beans, or any combination of those foods. You could even add some whole-grain bread or corn.

2. **Next, add lots of vegetables.**

   Choose from fresh, frozen, or canned veggies—the more the better.

3. **Then, add just a little protein for flavor and texture.**

    Remember, you don't need much protein to round out your meal. Just add a few slivers of beef, a sprinkle of tasty cheese, some ham strips, a dollop of ricotta, a tender chicken breast, a few slices of salmon, a couple of eggs, some tofu, or a handful of nuts. You can also find protein in grains and legumes.

4. **Think twice about using fat.**

    Check that you are using a healthy type of fat, either mono- or polyunsaturated. And use it sparingly.

Here are some low G.I. dinner ideas that your whole family will enjoy:

1. Team spaghetti bolognese with a green salad.
2. Wrap a fish fillet dressed with herbs and lemon, or tomato and onion, in foil and bake. Serve with a heavy-grain bread roll and salad.
3. Stir-fry chicken, meat, or fish with mixed green vegetables. Serve with brown rice or Chinese noodles.
4. Grill a steak and serve with a trio of low G.I. vegetables—sweet potato, corn, and peas.
5. Cook spinach and ricotta tortellini, team up with fresh garden vegetables and top with a tomato sauce.
6. Create a one-pot chicken casserole with your favorite vegetables, and chunks of baby new potatoes.
7. Make a lasagna—beef and cheese or vegetarian—and serve it with a crispy green salad of lettuce and celery and colorful pepper strips.

8. Buy a barbecued chicken, steam corn on the cob, and serve with a tossed salad.

9. Serve chili beans and beef with a soft tortilla bread or tacos and a salad.

10. Serve your favorite pasta (al dente) with a meat sauce or vegetable salsa, and couple it with lightly steamed green vegetables.

11. Cook a casserole using a good-quality chicken stock and chunks of your child's favorite vegetables, including sweet potatoes. Serve with brown rice or noodles.

12. Grill or barbecue a steak (or chicken or fish) and serve with a variety of low G.I. vegetables (sweet potatoes, corn, and peas) and crusty whole-grain rolls.

13. Stir-fry beef, chicken, or fish and serve with basmati rice or noodles.

14. Try a corn and green pea frittata, made with eggs and fresh vegetables or a can of corn and a small packet of frozen peas.

15. Bake Tex-Mex potatoes (sweet potatoes baked with onion, bacon, taco seasoning, baked beans, grated cheese, sour cream, and corn chips).

16. Serve grilled or barbecued sausages with corn on the cob and a 50–50 mixture of mashed new potatoes and mashed sweet potatoes.

17. Bake a tuna and rice casserole using Uncle Ben's Converted or brown rice, peas, corn, and strips of red pepper, topped with ½ cup of light cheese sauce made with skim or reduced fat milk.

18. Enjoy a risotto made with a low G.I. rice, lean meat, fish, or chicken and a variety of vegetables.

19. Buy one or two Chinese takeout stir-fry meals and split them with your family, padding them out with home-cooked low G.I. rice or pasta plus loads of vegetables.

Chapter 25

DESSERTS: A LOW G.I. FINISH

Children love desserts, which can add calcium and vitamin C to their meals if they're based on low fat dairy foods and fruits. Recipes incorporating fruit for sweetness will have more fiber and lower G.I. values than recipes with sugar. What's more, desserts are usually carbohydrate rich, which means they help us feel more full, and reduce the tendency for late night nibbles.

If you don't have time to prepare a dessert, try serving a bowl of in-season fruit or a fruit platter with cheese or yogurt. Remember, temperate-climate fruits such as apples, pears, peaches, citrus, and berries tend to have the lowest G.I. values.

For any of the following suggestions, you can substitute reduced fat milk or dairy products if you prefer.

QUICK AND EASY LOW G.I. DESSERTS

Almost everyone looks forward to a sweet, tasty dessert to top off a meal. Here are some simple ideas to end your meal in grand style.

1. Combine low fat ice cream and strawberries.
2. Bake apples whole, and stuff them with dried fruit or tapioca pudding.
3. Enjoy a fruit salad topped with low fat yogurt.
4. Make a fruit crisp: Top cooked fruit with a crumble mixture of oats, a little melted margarine (poly- or monounsaturated), and honey.
5. Slice a firm banana into some low fat custard.
6. Top canned fruit (peaches or pears) with low fat ice cream, low fat custard, or pudding.
7. Wrap sliced apple, raisins, nuts, and cinnamon in a sheet of phyllo pastry (brushed with milk, not fat) and bake as a strudel.
8. Make a winter fruit salad with segments of citrus fruits and raisins soaked in orange juice and honey.
9. Stew peaches or nectarines and serve them with low fat frozen yogurt.

Chapter 26

TAKEOUT FOODS

*Y*ou can make fairly healthy food choices at takeout restaurants if you keep some pointers in mind. Hint: Takeout foods that also happen to have a low G.I. value include fruit smoothies, ice cream, yogurt, popcorn, and some types of fresh fruit.

THE GLYCEMIC INDEX AND HEALTHY KIDS

TYPE OF TAKEOUT FOOD	BEST CHOICES	FOODS TO LIMIT
McDonald's, Burger King, or other hamburger outlets	Chunky chicken salad Small hamburger Chef salad (use low fat or fat-free dressing) Chicken tenders Plain ice cream cone Fruit	Deep-fried food Double meat Extra cheese Fried onion rings French fries Bacon Thick shakes Soft drinks
Pizza takeout/delivery Chinese takeout	Vegetarian topping Simple cheese topping Braised meat or chicken with steamed rice Stirfry vegetables or noodles	Pepperoni Double cheese topping Deep-fried egg or spring rolls or dim sum
Sandwich shops, delis, diners	Whole-grain roll or sandwich Veggie burger Grilled chicken salad or pita Milkshakes Frozen yogurt Ice cream or frozen yogurt	Pies Sausage rolls French fries Potato chips
Mexican restaurants such as Taco Bell	Bean burrito Chicken fajita Soft taco Beef taco Tostada with red sauce Frijoles and cheese	Nachos Crispy taco salads Refried beans Guacamole

Chapter 27

YOUR QUESTIONS ANSWERED

TRYING TODDLERS

My toddler refuses to eat most of the meals that I prepare. What can I do?

Welcome to the reality of the independent toddler! Refusing food is a normal part of toddler development. Usually it's not related to disliking a food, but rather is a way of exerting control. Don't be tempted to bribe your toddler with "treat" foods: Bribing, bullying, and fussing will only make the situation worse and reinforce poor eating habits. The best way to cope with food refusal is to try to avoid the whole situation in the first place. Toddlers need small meals and regular snacks, so allow yours to graze throughout the day as his or her appetite warrants; don't expect your toddler to eat set meals at set times. Expect the food intake to vary daily and use appetite as a guide to how much he or she needs. If you're still really concerned, keep a food diary for a week and include all the foods and fluids your toddler consumes—you may be surprised by how much he or she does eat! And if, after that, you're still worried, contact your doctor or dietitian for an individual assessment.

My toddler is so tired by the end of the day she won't eat her evening meal. What should I do?

It isn't unusual for tired toddlers to be uninterested in the evening meal; in fact, they can often be quite distracted if the whole family is sitting down together. Feeding toddlers earlier in the evening (5:00 or 5:30 P.M.) before fatigue sets in may help. Then they can sit with the family at the later mealtime without the pressure. If they consume more food during the family's evening meal, it's a bonus.

Another approach is to give toddlers their main meal at lunchtime when their appetites may be better. They can then be offered a lighter evening meal, such as sandwiches, fruit, or yogurt. Check the meal and snack suggestions on page 62 for ways to incorporate low G.I. foods into your child's usual food choices. A bottle or cup of milk before bed is a common bedtime routine in this age group and may help to satisfy your toddler's appetite for a longer period, since low G.I. foods such as milk make children feel fuller longer.

THE MEAL SKIPPERS

My daughter refuses to eat any breakfast before going to school. What should I do?

Breakfast is an important meal, so negotiate foods that she *will* eat—they don't necessarily need to be traditional breakfast foods. Check the breakfast list on page 62 for ideas. Your daughter may find two small low G.I. snacks (one at breakfast and one on the way to school) more acceptable.

My teenage daughter lives such a busy life with her studies, her friends, and a part-time job that she's always skipping meals. What should I do?

There is a tendency for many teens to skip meals or substitute less nutritious foods for nourishing meals, which may affect their health. Breakfast is the most commonly missed meal, particularly for girls. Research shows that skipping breakfast affects concentration levels at school or work and often causes teens to eat less nutritious mid-morning snacks because they are so intensely hungry. Dinner is another meal that teenagers commonly skip, often because of homework or social or sports commitments. It is important that teenagers take the time to eat regularly and sensibly. Plan some healthy low G.I. "heat and eat" snacks that your daughter can eat later in the day to help compensate for earlier missed meals, or make sure there are quick and easy low G.I. foods in the pantry that she can eat on the go.

My son eats so much after school that he's never hungry at dinnertime. What do you suggest?

If he's eating a lot of highly processed snack foods after school, such as chips, cookies, doughnuts, or high G.I. breakfast cereals (like Rice Krispies), then it is very likely he is eating too much of them, because these foods don't satisfy his appetite. Try providing some low G.I. foods that are more filling and harder to overeat. Great low G.I. snack choices include whole-grain sandwiches, fruit smoothies, fresh fruit, low G.I. breakfast cereals (such as Special K™) and yogurt. Check the low G.I. snack list on page 62 for other ideas. Increasing the amount of food in his lunch box and providing low G.I. food choices throughout the day may help too.

If he's eating because he's bored or simply sitting watching TV, encourage him to have his snack and then get involved in an out-of-school activity or sport.

SNACK SENSE

"Ravenous" hardly begins to describe my son when he comes home from school. What snack should I have ready for him?

The rapid growth spurt that occurs during puberty makes children's appetites increase significantly. Over a two- to-three-year period, boys can expect to gain eight inches in height and nine pounds in weight. Girls may gain six inches and seven pounds in height and weight respectively. It's essential that your son have a flexible meal schedule so that you can adapt it to these appetite fluctuations; the meals also have to be well-balanced in order to provide all the necessary nutrients for the growth spurt. Encourage your child to eat low G.I. foods during these appetite binges. Low G.I. foods tend to be more filling and so are better able to fill that bottomless pit and the hollow legs. Check the low G.I. snack and meal suggestions on page 62 for nutritious food ideas.

WEIGHTY CONCERN

My daughter is a little overweight for her age and height and is trying to diet. What can I do to help her?

It is quite natural for body fat levels to increase during the teen years. First you need to establish whether your daughter really is overweight, since it's not unusual for some teens to strive for an unrealistic weight below their healthy weight range.

If her weight gain is within the range of normal development, what she needs most from you is reassurance and strategies to build self-esteem and a positive body image. If your daughter *is* overweight, you need to consult a dietitian for an individual assessment so that a suitable long-term weight loss strategy can be tailored to meet her needs. (See page 105 to learn how to find a dietitian near you.)

Low G.I. foods may form part of this weight loss plan because they have some special advantages for people wanting to lose weight. They fill us up and keep us satisfied for longer, and they help us burn more fat and less muscle.

Becoming overweight is largely an imbalance between exercise and food intake, and both need to be addressed to achieve a healthy body weight. Eating low G.I. foods can help.

SUPPLEMENTAL ADVICE

Should I give my child a multivitamin supplement?

There is no clear benefit to supplementing the diet of well-nourished children with vitamins. As long as they eat a varied diet that contains the recommended number of servings from each of the five food groups,

THE GLYCEMIC INDEX AND HEALTHY KIDS

children's needs should be met. If you feel that your child's diet is inadequate, a multivitamin supplement taken as a quick fix won't solve the problem. First, a supplement isn't likely to compensate for all of the dietary inadequacies, and, second, you need to take great care to avoid overdosing on certain vitamins and minerals. It would be best to talk to your child's pediatrician or see a Registered Dietitian for advice. See page 105 for advice on finding a dietitian.

DAIRY DILEMMAS

My son loves milk, thank goodness, but he has a poor appetite, eats little else, and is constipated. What should I do?

Your son's love for milk may be the reason for his poor appetite. More than three to four servings a day (24 to 32 ounces) will detract from his appetite and prevent him from eating enough food from the other food groups, especially if the milk he's drinking is not low fat or skim. As a result, he may become constipated because of the lack of bulk or fiber in his gut and may suffer from other micronutrient deficiencies as well (such as iron deficiency, since milk contains no iron). Limit his dairy food intake to the recommended three or four servings a day and keep milk and other drinks separate from mealtimes to encourage his appetite. And if he's thirsty, there's nothing better than cold water. It's a good idea to keep a bottle in the fridge at all times.

My daughter refuses to drink milk. What can I do to change her mind?

Your daughter needs to have at least three servings a day of dairy foods to ensure that she's getting enough calcium. If she objects to plain milk, try flavoring it with one tablespoon of chocolate syrup or offer her hot cocoa. If she dislikes milk altogether, try offering other dairy foods, such as yogurt, ice cream, custard, or pudding. They're all great sources of calcium and excellent low G.I. food sources.

If she refuses all dairy foods, try a calcium-fortified soy alternative. Keep in mind that soy products don't contain naturally occurring calcium, as cow's milk does, so be sure to select only those brands that are adequately fortified with calcium (approximately 180 mg calcium per 4 ounces). If she also refuses soy products, you may need to consider a calcium supplement. We suggest that you consult your doctor or dietitian if she refuses all dairy and soy sources of calcium.

Chapter 28

HOW TO USE THE G.I. TABLES

The following table is an A to Z listing of the glycemic index values of commonly eaten foods in the United States and Canada. Approximately 300 different foods are listed, including some new values for foods tested only recently.

The glycemic index shown next to each food is the average for that food using glucose as the standard (i.e., glucose has a glycemic index of 100, with other foods rated accordingly). The average may represent the mean of 10 studies of that food worldwide or only two to four studies. In a few instances, American data is different from that of the rest of the world, and we show this data rather than the average. Rice and oatmeal fall into this category.

To check on a food's glycemic index, simply look

for it by name in the alphabetic list. You may also find it under a food type (e.g., fruit, cookies).

We've included in the tables the carbohydrate (CHO) and fat content of a sample serving of the food to help you keep track of the amount of fat and carbohydrate in your diet. The sample serving is not the recommended serving; it is just an example of a serving. The glycemic index does not depend on your serving size because it is a ranking of the glycemic effect of foods using carbohydrate-equivalent portion sizes. You can eat more of a low G.I. food or less of a high G.I. food and achieve the same blood sugar levels.

Remember that when you're choosing foods, the glycemic index isn't the only thing to consider: As far as blood sugar levels are concerned, you should also consider the amount of carbohydrate you are eating; for your overall health, the fat, fiber, and micronutrient content of your diet is also important. A dietitian can guide you further with good food choices; see page 105 for advice on finding a dietitian.

Chapter 29

THE GLYCEMIC INDEX TABLES

The G.I. values in these tables are correct at the time of publication. However, the formulation of some commercial foods can change, which can alter the glycemic index. Check our web page for revised and new data:
www.biochem.usyd.edu.au/~jennie/GI/glycemic_index.html

Note: You'll notice that certain foods have G.I. values exceeding 100. When measuring the glycemic index, experts use bread and glucose as the two reference foods, the standards against which the glycemic values of all other foods are measured. Glucose is used because it is the end product of digestion, and white bread is used because it is a staple in many of our diets. But foods with higher G.I. values do exist.

A–Z OF FOODS WITH GLYCEMIC INDEX, CARBOHYDRATE, AND FAT

Food	Glycemic Index	Fat (g per svg.)	CHO (g per svg.)
Agave nectar (90% fructose syrup), 1 tablespoon	11	0	12
All-Bran™, Kellogg's, breakfast cereal, ½ cup, 1 oz.	42 (av)	1	22
All-Bran with Extra Fiber™, Kellogg's, breakfast cereal, ½ cup, 1 oz.	51 (av)	1	2
Angel food cake, 1/12 cake, 1 oz.	67	trace	17
Apple, 1 medium, 5 ozs.	38 (av)	0	18
Apple, dried, 1 oz.	29	0	24
Apple juice, unsweetened, 1 cup, 8 ozs.	40	0	29
Apple cinnamon muffin, from mix, 1 muffin,	44	5	26
Apricots, fresh, 3 medium, 3 ozs.	57	0	12
canned, light syrup, 3 halves	64	0	14
dried, 5 halves	31	0	13
Apricot jam, no added sugar, 1 tablespoon	55	0	17
Apricot and honey muffin, low fat, from mix, 1 muffin	60	4	27
Arborio risotto rice, white, boiled, ⅔ cup	69	0	35
Bagel, 1 small, plain, 2 ozs.	72	1	38
Baked beans, ½ cup, 4 ozs.	48 (av)	1	24
Banana bread, 1 slice, 3 ozs.	47	7	46
Banana, raw, 1 medium, 5 ozs.	55 (av)	0	32
Banana, oat and honey muffin, low fat from mix, 1 muffin, small	65	4	27
Barley, pearled, boiled, ½ cup, 2.6 ozs.	25 (av)	0	22
Basmati white rice, boiled, 1 cup, 6 ozs.	58	0	50
Beans and legumes			
Baked beans, ½ cup, 4 ozs.	48 (av)	1	24
Black beans, boiled, ¾ cup, 4.3 ozs.	30	1	21
Black bean soup, ½ cup, 4½ ozs.	64	2	19
Blackeyed peas, canned, ½ cup, 4 ozs.	42	1	16
Broad beans, canned, ½ cup	79	1	9
Butter beans, boiled, ½ cup, 4 ozs.	31 (av)	0	16
Cannellini beans	31	0	16
Chickpeas (garbanzo beans),			
canned, drained, ½ cup, 4 ozs.	42	2	15
boiled, ½ cup, 3 ozs.	33 (av)	2	23

THE GLYCEMIC INDEX AND HEALTHY KIDS 91

Food	Glycemic Index	Fat (g per svg.)	CHO (g per svg.)
Fava beans, frozen, boiled, ½ cup, 3 ozs.	79	0	17
Green pea soup, canned, ready to serve, 1 cup, 9 ozs.	66	3	27
Kidney beans, red, boiled, ½ cup, 3 ozs.	27 (av)	0	20
Kidney beans, red, canned and drained, ½ cup, 4.3 ozs.	52	0	19
Lentils, green and brown, boiled, ½ cup, 3 ozs.	30 (av)	0	16
Lentils, red, boiled, 1.4 cup, 4 ozs.	26 (av)	0	27
Lentil soup, Unico, canned, 1 cup, 8 ozs.	44	1	24
Lima beans, baby, frozen, ½ cup, 3 ozs.	32	0	17
Mung beans, boiled, ½ cup, 3½ ozs.	38	1	18
Navy beans, boiled, ½ cup, 3 ozs.	38 (av)	0	19
Pea soup, split with ham, canned, 1 cup, 5 ½ ozs.	66	3	25
Peas, green, fresh, frozen, boiled, ½ cup, 2.7 ozs.	48 (av)	0	11
Peas dried, boiled, ½ cup, 2 ozs.	22	0	7
Pinto beans, canned, ½ cup, 4 ozs.	45	1	18
Pinto beans, soaked, boiled, ½ cup, 3 ozs.	39	0	22
Soy beans, boiled, ½ cup, 3 ozs.	18 (av)	7	10
Split peas, yellow, boiled, ½ cup, 3 ½ ozs.	32	0	21
Beets, canned, drained, ½ cup, 3 ozs.	64	0	5
Black bean soup, ½ cup, 4 ½ ozs.	64	2	19
Black beans, boiled, ¾ cup, 4.3 ozs.	30	1	21
Black bread, dark rye, 1 slice, 1.7 ozs.	76	1	18
Blackeyed peas, canned, ½ cup, 4 ozs.	42	1	16
Blueberry muffin, 1 muffin, 2 ozs.	59	4	27
Bran			
All-Bran with Extra Fiber™, Kellogg's, ½ cup, 1 oz	51	1	20
Bran Buds™, Kellogg's, ⅓ cup	58	1	14
Bran Flakes, Post, ⅔ cup, 1 oz.	74	1	22
Multi-Bran Chex™, General Mills, 1 cup, 2. ozs.	58	1.5	49
Oat bran, 1 tablespoon	55	1	7
Oat bran muffin, 2 ozs.	60	4	28
Rice bran, extruded, 1 tablespoon	19	2	3
Bran muffin, 1	60	8	34
Breads			
Dark rye, Black bread, 1 slice, 1.7 ozs.	76	1	18
Dark rye, Schinkenbröt, 1 slice, 2 ozs.	86	1	22
French baguette, 1 oz.	95	1	15

Food	Glycemic Index	Fat (g per svg.)	CHO (g per svg.)
Gluten-free bread, 1 slice, 1 oz.	90	1	18
Hamburger bun, 1 prepacked bun, 1½ ozs.	61	2	22
Kaiser roll, 1, 2 ozs.	73	2	34
Light deli (American) rye, 1 slice, 1 oz.	68	1	16
Melba toast, 6 pieces, 1 oz.	70	2	23
Pita bread, whole wheat, 6½ inch loaf, 2 ozs.	57	2	35
Pumpernickel, whole grain, 1 slice, 1 oz.	51	1	16
Rye bread, 1 slice, 1 oz.	65	1	15
Sourdough, 1 slice, 1½ ozs.	52	1	20
Natural Ovens 100% Whole Grain, 1 slice, 1.2 ozs.	51	0	17
Natural Ovens Hunger Filler, 1 slice, 1.2 ozs.	59	0	16
Natural Ovens Natural Wheat, 1 slice, 1.2 ozs.	59	0	16
Natural Ovens Happiness, 1 slice, 1.1 ozs.	63	0	15
Sourdough rye, Arnold's, 1 slice, 1½ ozs.	57	1	21
White, 1 slice, 1 oz.	70 (av)	1	12
100% stoneground whole wheat, 1 slice, 1½ ozs.	53	1	12
Whole wheat, 1 slice, 1 oz.	69 (av)	1	13
Bread stuffing from mix, 2 ozs.	74	5	13
Breakfast cereals			
All-Bran™, Kellogg's, breakfast cereal, ½ cup, 1 oz.	42 (av)	1	22
All-Bran with Extra Fiber™, Kellogg's, ½ cup, 1 oz.	51	1	20
Bran Buds™, Kellogg's, ⅓ cup	58	1	14
Bran Flakes, Post, ⅔ cup, 1 oz.	74	1	22
Cheerios™, General Mills, 1 cup, 1 oz.	74	2	23
Cocoa Krispies™, Kellogg's, 1 cup, 1 oz.	77	1	27
Corn Bran™, Quaker Crunchy, ¾ cup, 1 oz.	75	1	23
Corn Chex™, Nabisco, 1 cup, 1 oz.	83	0	26
Corn Flakes™, Kellogg's, 1 cup, 1 oz.	84 (av)	0	24
Corn Pops™, 1 cup	80	0	27
Cream of Wheat, instant, 1 packet, 1 oz.	74	0	21
Cream of Wheat, old fashioned, ¾ cup, cooked, 6 ozs.	66	0	21
Crispix™, Kellogg's, 1 cup, 1 oz.	87	0	25
Frosted Flakes™, Kellogg's, ¾ cup, 1 oz.	55	0	28
Golden Grahams™, General Mills, ¾ cup, 1.6 ozs.	71	1	25
Grapenuts™, Post, ½ cup, 1 oz.	71	1	47
Grapenuts Flakes™, Post, ¾ cup, 1 oz.	80	1	24
Just Right™, ¾ cup	60	1	36

THE GLYCEMIC INDEX AND HEALTHY KIDS 93

Food	Glycemic Index	Fat (g per svg.)	CHO (g per svg.)
Life™, Quaker, ¾ cup, 1 oz.	66	1	25
Mini Wheats (whole wheat), 1 cup	58	0	21
Muesli, natural muesli, ⅔ cup, 1½ ozs.	56	3	28
Muesli, breakfast cereal, toasted, ⅔ cup, 2 ozs.	43	3	41
Multi-Bran Chex™, General Mills, 1 cup, 2. ozs.	58	1.5	49
Nutri-grain™ breakfast cereal, 1 cup	66	0	20
Oat bran, raw, 1 tablespoon	55	1	7
Oat bran™, Quaker Oats, breakfast cereal, ¾ cup, 1 oz.	50	1	23
Oatmeal (made with water), old fashioned, cooked, ½ cup, 4 ozs.	49 (av)	1	12
Oats, 1-minute, Quaker Oats, 1 cup, cooked	66	2	25
Puffed Wheat™, Quaker, 2 cups, 1 oz.	80	0	22
Raisin Bran™, Kellogg's, ¾ cup, 1 oz.	73	0	32
Rice bran, 1 tablespoon	19	2	5
Rice Chex™, General Mills, 1¼ cups, 1 oz.	89	0	27
Rice Krispies™, Kellogg's, 1¼ cups, 1 oz.	82	0	26
Shredded Wheat™, Post, breakfast cereal, ½ cup, 1 oz.	83	1	23
Shredded wheat, 1 biscuit, ⅘ oz.	62	0	19
Shredded wheat, spoonsize, ⅔ cup, 1.2 ozs.	58	0	27
Smacks™, Kellogg's, ¾ cup, 1 oz.	56	1	27
Special K™, Kellogg's, 1 cup, 1 oz.	54	0	22
Team Flakes™, Nabisco, ¾ cup, 1 oz.	82	0	25
Total™, General Mills, ¾ cup, 1 oz.	76	1	24
WeetaBix™, 2 biscuits, 1.2 ozs.	75	1	28
Breton wheat crackers, 6	67	6	14
Broad beans, canned, ½ cup	79	1	9
Buckwheat groats, cooked, ½ cup, 2.7 ozs.	54 (av)	1	20
Bulgur, cooked, ⅔ cup, 4 ozs.	48 (av)	0	23
Bun, hamburger, 1 prepacked bun, 1.7 ozs.	61	2	22
Butter beans, boiled, ½ cup, 4 ozs.	31 (av)	0	16
Cakes			
Angel food cake, 1 slice, 1/12 cake, 1 oz.	67	trace	17
Banana bread, 1 slice, 3 ozs.	47	7	46
Chocolate fudge cake, pkt. mix, with dark Dutch fudge frosting, Betty Crocker, 1/12 of cake, with 2 tablespoons frosting	38	17	54
French vanilla cake, pkt. mix, with vanilla frosting, Betty Crocker, 1/12 of cake, with 2 tablespoons frosting	42	15	58

THE GLUCOSE REVOLUTION POCKET GUIDE

Food	Glycemic Index	Fat (g per svg.)	CHO (g per svg.)
Pound cake, homemade, 1 slice, 3 ozs.	54	15	42
Sponge cake, 1 slice, 1/12 cake, 2 ozs.	46	4	32
Capellini pasta, cooked, 1 cup, 6 ozs.	45	1	53
Cannellini beans, boiled, 1/2 cup, 4 ozs.	31	0	16
Cantaloupe, raw, 1/4 small, 6 1/2 ozs.	65	0	16
Carrots, peeled, boiled, 1/2 cup, 2.4 ozs.	49	0	3
Cereal grains			
Barley, pearled, boiled, 1/2 cup, 2.6 ozs.	25 (av)	0	22
Bulgur, cooked, 1/2 cup, 3 ozs.	48 (av)	0	17
Couscous, cooked, 1/2 cup, 3 ozs.	65 (av)	0	21
Corn			
Cornmeal, whole grain, from mix, cooked, 1/3 cup, 1.4 ozs.	68	1	30
Corn, canned, drained, 1/2 cup, 3 ozs.	55 (av)	1	15
Taco shells, 2 shells, 1 oz.	68	5	17
Rice			
Basmati, white, boiled, 1 cup, 6 ozs.	58	0	50
Brown, 1 cup, 6 ozs.	55 (av)	0	37
Converted™, Uncle Ben's, 1 cup, 6 ozs.	44	38	
Instant, cooked, 1 cup, 6 ozs.	87	0	37
Long grain, white, 1 cup, 6 ozs.	56 (av)	0	42
Parboiled, 1 cup, 6 ozs.	48	0	38
Rice cakes, plain, 3 cakes, 1 oz.	82	1	23
Short grain, white, 1 cup, 6 ozs.	72	0	42
Chana dal, 1/2 cup, 4 ozs.	8	3	28
Cheerios™, General Mills, breakfast cereal, 1 cup, 1 oz.	74	2	23
Cherries, 10 large cherries, 3 ozs.	22	0	10
Chickpeas (garbanzo beans),			
canned, drained, 1/2 cup, 4 ozs.	42	2	15
boiled, 1/2 cup, 3 ozs.	33 (av)	2	23
Chocolate butterscotch muffin, low fat from mix, 1 muffin	53	4	28
Chocolate, bar, 1 1/2 ozs.	49	14	26
Chocolate Flavor, Nestle Quik™ (made with water), 3 teaspoons	53	0	14
Chocolate fudge cake, pkt. mix, with dark Dutch fudge frosting, Betty Crocker, 1/12 of cake, with 2 tablespoons frosting	38	17	54
Coca-Cola™, soft drink, 1 can	63	0	41
Cocoa Krispies™, Kellogg's, breakfast cereal, 1 cup, 1 oz.	77	1	27

THE GLYCEMIC INDEX AND HEALTHY KIDS

Food	Glycemic Index	Fat (g per svg.)	CHO (g per svg.)
Corn			
Cornmeal (polenta), 1/3 cup, 1.4 ozs.	68	1	30
Corn, canned and drained, 1/2 cup, 3 ozs.	55 (av)	1	15
Corn Bran™, Quaker Crunchy, breakfast cereal, 3/4 cup, 1 oz.	75	1	23
Corn Chex™, General Mills, breakfast cereal, 1 cup, 1 oz.	83	0	
Corn chips, 1 oz.	72	10	16
Corn Flakes™, Kellogg's, breakfast cereal, 1 cup, 1 oz.	84 (av)	0	24
Corn Pops™, 1 cup	80	0	27
Cornmeal, from mix, cooked, 1/3 cup, 1.4 ozs.	68	1	30
Cookies			
Graham crackers, 4 squares, 1 oz.	74	3	22
Milk Arrowroot, 3 cookies, 1/2 oz.	69	2	9
Oatmeal, 1 cookie, 2/3 oz.	55	3	12
Shortbread, 4 small cookies, 1 oz.	64	7	19
Social Tea™ biscuits, Nabisco, 4 cookies, 2/3 oz.	55	3	13
Vanilla wafers, 7 cookies, 1 oz.	77	4	21
see also Crackers			
Couscous, cooked, 2/3 cup, 4 ozs.	65 (av)	0	21
Crackers			
Breton wheat crackers, 6	67	6	14
Crispbread, 3 crackers, 2/3 oz.	81	0	15
Kavli™ All Natural Whole Grain Crispbread, 4 wafers, 1 oz.	71	1	16
Premium saltine crackers, 8 crackers, 1 oz.	74	3	17
Rice cakes, plain, 3 cakes, 1 oz.	82	1	23
Ryvita™ Tasty Dark Rye Whole Grain Crisp Bread, 2 slices, 2/3 oz.	69	1	16
Stoned wheat thins, 3 crackers, 4/5 oz.	67	2	15
Water cracker, Carr's, 3 king size crackers, 4/5 oz.	78	2	18
Cranberry juice cocktail, 8 ozs.	52	0	31
Cream of Wheat, instant, 1 packet, 1 oz.	74	0	21
Cream of Wheat, old fashioned, 3/4 cup, cooked, 6 ozs.	66	0	21
Crispix™, Kellogg's, breakfast cereal, 1 cup, 1 oz.	87	0	25
Croissant, medium, 1.2 ozs.	67	14	27
Cupcake, with icing and cream filling, 1 cake	73	3	26
Custard, 3/4 cup, 4.4 ozs.	43	5	36
Dairy foods and nondairy substitutes			
Ice cream, 10% fat, vanilla, 1/2 cup, 2.2 ozs.	61 (av)	7	16

96 THE GLUCOSE REVOLUTION POCKET GUIDE

Food	Glycemic Index	Fat (G per svg.)	CHO (G per svg.)
Ice milk, vanilla, ½ cup, 2.2 ozs.	50	3	15
Milk, whole, 1 cup, 8 ozs.	27 (av)	9	11
skim, 1 cup, 8 ozs.	32	0	12
chocolate flavored, 1%, 1 cup, 8 ozs.	34	3	26
Pudding, ½ cup, 4.4 ozs.	43	4	27
Soy milk, 1 cup, 8 ozs.	31	7	14
Tofu frozen dessert (nondairy), low fat, ½ cup, 2 ozs.	115	1	21
Yogurt			
nonfat, fruit flavored, with sugar, 8 ozs.	33	0	30
nonfat, plain, artificial sweetener, 8 ozs.	14	0	17
nonfat, fruit flavored, artificial sweetener, 8 ozs.	14	0	17
Dates, dried, 5, 1.4 ozs.	103	0	27
Doughnut with cinnamon and sugar, 1.6 ozs.	76	11	29
Fanta™, soft drink, 1 can	68	0	47
Fava beans, frozen, boiled, ½ cup, 3 ozs.	79	0	17
Fettucine, cooked, 1 cup, 6 ozs.	32	1	57
Fish sticks, frozen, oven-cooked, fingers, 3½ sticks	38	14	24
Flan (creme caramel), ½ cup, 4 ozs.	65	5	23
French baguette bread, 1 oz., about one 1-inch slice	95	0	15
French fries, large, 4.3 ozs.	75	22	46
French vanilla cake, pkt. mix, with vanilla frosting, Betty Crocker, ¹⁄₁₂ of cake, with 2 tablespoons frosting	42	15	58
Frosted Flakes™, Kellogg's, breakfast cereal, ¾ cup, 1 oz.	55	0	28
Fructose, pure, 3 packets	23 (av)	0	10
Fruit cocktail, canned in natural juice, ½ cup, 4 ozs.	55	0	15
Fruits and fruit products			
Agave nectar (90% fructose syrup), 1 tablespoon	11	0	12
Apple, 1 medium, 5 ozs.	38 (av)	0	18
Apple, dried, 1 oz.	29	0	24
Apple juice, unsweetened, 1 cup, 8 ozs.	40	0	29
Apricots, fresh, 3 medium, 3.3 ozs.	57	0	12
canned, light syrup, 3 halves	64	0	19
dried, 1 oz.	31	0	13
Apricot jam, no added sugar, 1 tablespoon	55	0	17
Banana, raw, 1 medium, 5 ozs.	55 (av)	0	32
Cherries, 10 large, 3 ozs.	22	0	10
Cranberry juice cocktail, 8 ozs.	52	0	31

Food	Glycemic Index	Fat (g per svg.)	CHO (g per svg.)
Dates, dried, 5, 1.4 ozs.	103	0	27
Fruit cocktail, canned in natural juice, ½ cup, 4 ozs.	55	0	15
Grapefruit, raw, ½ medium, 3.3 ozs.	25	0	5
Grapefruit juice, unsweetened, 1 cup, 8 ozs.	48	0	22
Grapes, green, 1 cup, 3 ozs.	46 (av)	0	15
Kiwi, 1 medium, raw, peeled, 2½ ozs.	52 (av)	0	8
Lychee, canned and drained, 7	79	0	16
Mango, 1 small, 5 ozs.	55 (av)	0	19
Marmalade, 1 tablespoon	48	0	17
Orange, navel, 1 medium, 4 ozs.	44 (av)	0	10
Orange juice, 1 cup, 8 ozs.	46	0	26
Papaya, ½ medium, 5 ozs.	58 (av)	0	14
Peach, fresh, 1 medium, 3 ozs.	30	0	7
canned, natural juice, ½ cup, 4 ozs.	30	0	14
canned, light syrup, ½ cup, 4 ozs.	52	0	18
canned, heavy syrup, ½ cup, 4 ozs.	58	0	26
Pear, fresh, 1 medium, 5 ozs.	38 (av)	0	21
canned in pear juice, ½ cup, 4 ozs.	44	0	13
Pineapple, fresh, 2 slices, 4 ozs.	66	0	10
Pineapple juice, unsweetened, canned, 8 ozs.	46	0	34
Plums, 1 medium, 2 ozs.	39 (av)	0	7
Prunes, pitted, 6	29	0	25
Raisins, ¼ cup, 1 oz.	64	0	28
Strawberry jam, 1 tablespoon	51	0	18
Watermelon, 1 cup, 5 ozs.	72	0	8
Gatorade™ sports drink, 1 cup, 8 ozs.	78	0	14
Glucose powder, 2½ tablets	102	0	10
Gluten-free bread, 1 slice, 1 oz.	90	1	18
Glutinous rice, white, steamed, 1 cup	98	0	37
Gnocchi, cooked, 1 cup, 5 ozs.	68	3	71
Golden Grahams™, General Mills, ¾ cup, 1.6 ozs.	71	1	25
Graham crackers, 4 squares, 1 oz.	74	3	22
Granola Bars™, Quaker Chewy, 1 oz.	61	2	23
Grapefruit, raw, ½ medium, 3.3 ozs.	25	0	5
Grapefruit juice unsweetened, 1 cup, 8 ozs.	48	0	22
Grapenuts™, Post, breakfast cereal, ½ cup, 1 oz.	71	1	47
Grapenuts Flakes™, Post, breakfast cereal, ¾ cup, 1 oz.	80	1	24

Food	Glycemic Index	Fat (g per svg.)	CHO (g per svg.)
Grapes, green, 1 cup, 3.3 ozs.	46 (av)	0	15
Green pea soup, canned, ready to serve, 1 cup, 9 ozs.	66	3	27
Hamburger bun, 1 prepacked bun, 1½ ozs.	61	2	22
Honey, 1 tablespoon	58	0	16
Ice cream, 10% fat, vanilla, ½ cup, 2.2 ozs.	61 (av)	7	16
Ice milk, vanilla, ½ cup, 2.2 ozs.	50	3	15
Isostar, 1 cup, 8 ozs.	70	0	18
Jasmine, white, long grain, steamed, 1 cup	109	0	39
Jelly beans, 10 large, 1 oz.	80	0	26
Just Right™, breakfast cereal, ¾ cup	60	1	36
Kaiser rolls, 1 roll, 2 ozs.	73	2	34
Kavli™ All Natural Whole Grain Crispbread, 4 wafers, 1 oz.	71	1	16
Kidney beans, red, boiled, ½ cup, 3 ozs.	27 (av)	0	20
Kidney beans, red, canned and drained, ½ cup, 4.3 ozs.	52	0	19
Kiwi, 1 medium, raw, peeled, 2½ ozs.	52 (av)	0	8
Kudos Granola Bars™ (whole grain), 1 bar, 1 oz.	62	5	20
Lactose, pure, ⁷⁄₁₀ oz.	46 (av)	0	10
Lentil soup, Unico, canned, 1 cup, 8 ozs.	44	1	24
Lentils, green and brown, boiled, ½ cup, 3 ozs.	30 (av)	0	16
Lentils, red, boiled, 1.4 cup, 4 ozs.	26 (av)	0	27
Life™, Quaker, breakfast cereal, ¾ cup, 1 oz.	66	1	25
Life Savers™, roll candy, 6 pieces, peppermint	70	0	10
Light deli (American) rye bread, 1 slice, 1 oz.	68	1	16
Lima beans, baby, frozen, ½ cup, 3 ozs.	32	0	17
Linguine pasta, thick, cooked, 1 cup, 6 ozs.	46 (av)	1	56
Linguine pasta, thin, cooked, 1 cup, 6 ozs.	55 (av)	1	56
Lychee, canned and drained, 7	79	0	16
M&M's Chocolate Candies Peanut™, 1.7 oz. package	33	13	30
Macaroni and Cheese Dinner™, Kraft packaged, cooked, 1 cup, 7 ozs.	64	17	48
Macaroni, cooked, 1 cup, 6 ozs.	45	1	42
Maltose (maltodextrin), pure, 2½ teaspoons	105	0	10
Mango, 1 small, 5 ozs.	55 (av)	0	19
Marmalade, 1 tablespoon	48	0	17
Mars Almond Bar™, 1.8 ozs.	65	12	31
Mars Bar™, 1 bar	65	11	41
Melba toast, 6 pieces, 1 oz.	70	1	23

Food	Glycemic Index	Fat (g per svg.)	CHO (g per svg.)
Milk, whole, 1 cup, 8 ozs.	27 (av)	9	11
skim, 1 cup, 8 ozs.	32	0	12
chocolate flavored, 1%, 1 cup, 8 ozs.	34	3	26
Milk Arrowroot, 3 cookies, ½ oz.	63	2	9
Millet, cooked, ½ cup, 4 ozs.	71	1	28
Mini Wheats (whole wheat), breakfast cereal, 1 cup	58	0	21
Muesli, breakfast cereal, toasted, ⅔ cup, 2 ozs.	43	3	41
Muesli, non-toasted, ⅔ cup, 1½ ozs.	56	3	28
Multi-Bran Chex™, General Mills, 1 cup, 2. ozs.	58	1.5	49
Muffins			
Apple cinnamon, from mix, 1 muffin, 2 ozs.	44	8	33
Apricot and honey, low fat, from mix, 1 muffin	60	4	27
Banana, oat and honey, low fat, from mix, 1 muffin, small	65	4	28
Blueberry, 1 muffin, 2 ozs.	59	4	27
Bran, 1 muffin	60	8	34
Chocolate butterscotch, low fat, from mix, 1 muffin	53	4	28
Oat and raisin, low fat, from mix, 1 muffin	54	3	28
Oat bran, 1 muffin, 2 ozs.	60	4	28
Mung beans, boiled, ½ cup, 3½ ozs.	38	1	18
Mung bean noodles, 1 cup	39	0	35
Natural Ovens 100% Whole Grain bread, 1 slice, 1.2 ozs.	51	0	17
Natural Ovens Hunger Filler bread, 1 slice, 1.2 ozs.	59	0	16
Natural Ovens Natural Wheat bread, 1 slice, 1.2 ozs.	59	0	16
Natural Ovens Happiness bread, 1 slice, 1.1 ozs.	63	0	15
Navy beans, boiled, ½ cup, 3 ozs.	38 (av)	0	19
Noodles, mung bean, 1 cup	39	0	35
Nutella™ (spread), 2 tablespoons	33	9	19
Nutri-grain™ breakfast cereal, 1 cup	66	0	20
Oat and raisin muffin, low fat from mix, 1 muffin	54	3	28
Oat bran, 1 tablespoon	55	1	7
Oat bran™, Quaker Oats, breakfast cereal, ¾ cup, 1 oz.	50	1	23
Oat bran, 1 muffin, 2 ozs.	60	4	28
Oatmeal (made with water), old fashioned, cooked, ½ cup, 4 ozs.	49	1	12
Oatmeal cookie, 1, ⅖ oz.	55	3	12
Oats, 1-minute, Quaker Oats, 1 cup, cooked	66	2	25
Orange, navel, 1 medium, 4 ozs.	44 (av)	0	10

THE GLUCOSE REVOLUTION POCKET GUIDE

Food	Glycemic Index	Fat (g per svg.)	CHO (g per svg.)
Orange syrup, diluted, 1 cup	66	0	20
Orange juice, 1 cup, 8 ozs.	46	0	26
Papaya, ½ medium, 5 ozs.	58 (av)	0	14
Parsnips, boiled, ½ cup, 2½ ozs.	97	0	15
Pasta			
Capellini, cooked, 1 cup, 6 ozs.	45	1	53
Fettuccine, cooked, 1 cup, 6 ozs.	32	1	57
Gnocchi, cooked, 1 cup, 5 ozs.	68	3	71
Linguine thick, cooked, 1 cup, 6 ozs.	46 (av)	1	56
Linguine thin, cooked, 1 cup, 6 ozs.	55 (av)	1	56
Macaroni, cooked, 1 cup, 5 ozs.	45	1	42
Macaroni & Cheese Dinner™, Kraft, packaged, cooked, 1 cup, 7 ozs.	64	17	48
Ravioli, meat-filled, cooked, 4 large	39	6	41
Spaghetti, white, cooked, 1 cup, 6 ozs.	41 (av)	1	42
Spaghetti, whole wheat, cooked, 1 cup, 6 ozs.	37 (av)	1	48
Spirali, durum, cooked, 1 cup, 6 ozs.	43	1	56
Star Pastina, cooked, 1 cup, 6 ozs.	38	1	56
Tortellini, cheese, cooked, 8 ozs.	50	7	28
Vermicelli, cooked, 1 cup, 6 ozs.	35	0	42
Pastry, flaky, ⅛ of double crust, 2 ozs.	59	15	24
Pea soup, split with ham, canned, 1 cup, 5½ ozs.	66	3	25
Peach, fresh, 1 medium, 3 ozs.	30	0	7
canned, heavy syrup, ½ cup, 4 ozs.	58	0	26
canned, light syrup, ½ cup, 4 ozs.	52	0	18
canned, natural juice, ½ cup, 4 ozs.	30	0	14
Peanuts, roasted, salted, ½ cup, 1.1 oz. bag	15 (av)	38	7
Pear, fresh, 1 medium, 5 ozs.	38 (av)	0	21
canned in pear juice, ½ cup, 4 ozs.	44	0	13
Peas, green, fresh, frozen, boiled, ½ cup, 2.7 ozs.	48 (av)	0	10
Peas dried, boiled, ½ cup, 2 ozs.	22	0	12
Pineapple, fresh, 2 slices, 4 ozs.	66	0	10
Pineapple juice, unsweetened, canned, 8 ozs.	46	0	34
Pinto beans, canned, ½ cup, 4 ozs.	45	1	18
Pinto beans, soaked, boiled, ½ cup, 3 ozs.	39	0	22
Pita bread, whole wheat, 6½ inch loaf, 2 ozs.	57	2	35

THE GLYCEMIC INDEX AND HEALTHY KIDS 101

Food	Glycemic Index	Fat (g per svg.)	CHO (g per svg.)
Pizza, cheese and tomato, 2 slices, 8 ozs.	60	22	56
Pizza, Super Supreme, Pizza Hut, pan, 2 slices	36	31	72
Pizza, Super Supreme, Pizza Hut, thin and crispy, 2 slices	30	27	50
Plums, 1 medium, 2 ozs.	39 (av)	0	7
Popcorn, light, microwave, 1¾ oz. snack size	55	8	30
Pop Tarts™, double chocolate, 1 tart	70	5	36
Potatoes			
Desirée, peeled, boiled, 1 medium, 4 ozs.	101	0	13
French fries, large, 4.3 ozs.	75	26	49
instant mashed potatoes, Carnation Foods™, ½ cup, 3½ ozs.	86	2	14
new, unpeeled, boiled, 4 medium, 6 ozs.	78 (av)	0	25
new, canned, drained, 5 small, 6 ozs.	61	0	26
red-skinned, peeled, boiled, 1 medium, 4 ozs.	88 (av)	0	15
red-skinned, baked in oven (no fat), 1 medium, 4 ozs.	93 (av)	0	15
red-skinned, mashed, ½ cup, 4 ozs.	91 (av)	0	16
red-skinned, microwaved, 1 medium, 4 ozs.	79	0	15
sweet potato, peeled, boiled, mashed, ½ cup 3 ozs.	54 (av)	0	20
white-skinned, peeled, boiled, 1 medium, 4 ozs.	63 (av)	0	24
white-skinned, with skin, baked in oven (no fat), 1 medium, 4 ozs.	85 (av)	0	30
white-skinned, mashed, ½ cup, 4 ozs.	70 (av)	0	20
white-skinned, with skin, microwaved, 1 medium, 4 ozs.	82	0	29
Sebago, peeled, boiled, 1 medium, 4 ozs.	87	0	13
Potato chips, plain, 14 pieces, 1 oz.	54 (av)	10	15
Pound cake, 1 slice, homemade, 3 ozs.	54	15	42
Power Bar™, Performance, Chocolate, 1 bar	58	2	45
Premium saltine crackers, 8 crackers, 1 oz.	74	3	17
Pretzels, 1 oz.	83	1	22
Prunes, pitted, 6	29	0	25
Puffed Wheat™, Quaker, breakfast cereal, 2 cups, 1 oz.	80	0	22
Pumpernickel bread, whole grain, 2 slices	51	2	32
Pumpkin, peeled, boiled, mashed, ½ cup, 4 ozs.	75	0	6
Raisins, ¼ cup, 1 oz.	64	0	28
Raisin Bran™, Kellogg's, breakfast cereal, ¾ cup, 1.3 ozs.	73	0	32
Ravioli, meat-filled, cooked, 4 large	39	6	41

Food	Glycemic Index	Fat (g per svg.)	CHO (g per svg.)
Rice			
Arborio risotto rice, white, boiled, ⅔ cup	69	0	35
Basmati, white, boiled, 1 cup, 7 ozs.	58	0	50
Brown, 1 cup, 6 ozs.	55 (av)	0	37
Converted™, Uncle Ben's, 1 cup, 6 ozs.	44	0	38
Glutinous, white, steamed, 1 cup	98	0	37
Instant, cooked, 1 cup, 6 ozs.	87	0	38
Jasmine, white, long grain, steamed, 1 cup	109	0	39
Long grain, white, 1 cup, 6 ozs.	56 (av)	0	42
Parboiled, extruded, 1 cup, 6 ozs.	48	0	38
Rice bran, 1 tablespoon	19	2	3
Rice cakes, plain, 3 cakes, 1 oz.	82	1	23
Short grain, white, 1 cup, 6 ozs.	72	0	42
Rice Chex™, General Mills, breakfast cereal, 1¼ cups, 1 oz.	89	0	27
Rice Krispies™, Kellogg's, breakfast cereal, 1¼ cups, 1 oz.	82	0	26
Rice vermicelli, cooked, 6 ozs.	58	0	48
Roll (bread), Kaiser, 1 roll, 2 ozs.	73	2	39
Roll-ups™, 1 fruit leather	99	1	13
Romano (cranberry) beans, boiled, ½ cup, 3 ozs.	46	0	21
Rutabaga, peeled, boiled, ½ cup, 2.6 ozs.	72	0	3
Rye bread, 1 slice, 1 oz.	65	1	15
Ryvita™ Tasty Dark Rye Whole Grain Crisp Bread, 2 slices, ⅔ oz.	69	1	16
Semolina, cooked, ⅔ cup, 6 ozs.	55	0	17
Shortbread, 4 small cookies, 1 oz.	64	7	19
Shredded Wheat™, Post, breakfast cereal, 1 oz.	83	1	23
Shredded wheat, 1 biscuit, ⅘ oz.	62	0	19
Shredded wheat, spoonsize, 1 cup, 1.2 ozs.	58	0	27
Skittles Original Fruit Bite Size Candies™, 2.3 oz. pk.	70	3	59
Smacks™, Kellogg's, breakfast cereal, ¾ cup, 1 oz.	56	1	27
Snickers™, 2.2 oz. bar	41	15	36
Social Tea™ biscuits, Nabisco, 4 cookies, ⅔ oz.	55	3	13
Soft drink, Coca-Cola™, 1 can, 12 ozs.	63	0	39
Soft drink, Fanta™, 1 can, 12 ozs.	68	0	47
Soups			
Black bean soup, ½ cup, 4½ ozs.	64	2	19
Green pea soup, canned, ready to serve, 1 cup, 9 ozs.	66	3	27

THE GLYCEMIC INDEX AND HEALTHY KIDS

Food	Glycemic Index	Fat (g per svg.)	CHO (g per svg.)
Lentil soup, Unico, canned, 1 cup, 8 ozs.	44	1	24
Pea soup, split with ham, 1 cup, 5½ ozs.	66	3	25
Tomato soup, canned, 1 cup, 9 ozs.	38	4	33
Sourdough bread, 1 slice, 1½ ozs.	52	1	20
Rye bread, Arnold's, 1 slice, 1½ ozs.	57	1	21
Soy beans, boiled, ½ cup, 3 ozs.	18 (av)	7	10
Soy milk, 1 cup, 8 ozs.	31	7	14
Spaghetti, white, cooked, 1 cup	41 (av)	1	42
Spaghetti, whole wheat, cooked, 1 cup, 5 ozs.	37 (av)	1	48
Special K™, Kellogg's, breakfast cereal, 1 cup, 1 oz.	54	0	22
Spirali, durum, cooked, 1 cup, 6 ozs.	43	1	56
Split pea soup, 8 ozs.	60	4	38
Split peas, yellow, boiled, ½ cup, 3½ ozs.	32	0	29
Sponge cake plain, 1 slice, 3½ ozs.	46	4	32
Sports drinks			
Gatorade™ 1 cup, 8 ozs.	78	0	14
Isostar, 1 cup, 8 ozs.	70	0	18
Sportsplus, 1 cup, 8 ozs.	74	0	17
Power Bar™, Performance Chocolate Bar, 1 bar	58	3	45
Stoned wheat thins, 3 crackers, ⅘ oz.	67	2	15
Strawberry Nestle Quik™ (made with water), 3 teaspoons	64	0	14
Strawberry jam, 1 tablespoon	51	0	18
Sucrose, 1 teaspoon	65 (av)	0	4
Super Supreme pizza, Pizza Hut, pan, 2 slices	36	31	72
Super Supreme pizza, Pizza Hut, thin and crispy, 2 slices	30	27	50
Syrup, fruit flavored, diluted, 1 cup	66	0	20
Sweet potato, peeled, boiled, mashed, ½ cup 3 ozs.	54 (av)	0	20
Taco shells, 2 shells, 1 oz.	68	5	17
Tapioca pudding, boiled with whole milk, 1 cup, 10 ozs.	81	13	51
Taro, peeled, boiled, ½ cup, 2 ozs.	54	0	23
Team Flakes™, Nabisco, breakfast cereal, ¾ cup, 1 oz.	82	0	25
Tofu frozen dessert, nondairy, low fat, 2 ozs.	115	1	21
Tomato soup, canned, 1 cup, 9 ozs.	38	4	33
Tortellini, cheese, cooked, 8 ozs.	50	7	28
Total™, General Mills, breakfast cereal, ¾ cup, 1 oz.	76	1	24
Twix Chocolate Caramel Cookie™, 2, 2 ozs.	44	14	37
Vanilla wafers, 7 cookies, 1 oz.	77	4	21

Food	Glycemic Index	Fat (g per svg.)	CHO (g per svg.)
Vermicelli, cooked, 1 cup, 6 ozs.	35	0	42
Vitasoy™ Soy milk, creamy original, 1 cup, 8 ozs.	31	7	14
Waffles, plain, frozen, 4 inch square, 1 oz.	76	3	13
Water crackers, 3 king size crackers, ⅘ oz.	78	2	18
Watermelon, 1 cup, 5 ozs.	72	0	8
Weetabix™ breakfast cereal, 2 biscuits, 1.2 ozs.	75	1	28
White bread, 1 slice, 1 oz.	70 (av)	1	12
Whole wheat bread, 1 slice, 1 oz.	69 (av)	1	13
Yam, boiled, 3 ozs.	51	0	24
Yogurt			
nonfat, fruit flavored, with sugar, 8 ozs.	33	0	30
nonfat, plain, artificial sweetener, 8 ozs.	14	0	17
nonfat, fruit flavored, artificial sweetener, 8 ozs.	14	0	17

FOR MORE INFORMATION

*I*f you'd like to know the glycemic index of more foods, write to the food manufacturers and encourage them to contact:

SYDNEY UNIVERSITY GLYCEMIC INDEX RESEARCH SERVICE (SUGIRS)

Dr. Jennie Brand-Miller
Department of Biochemistry
University of Sydney
NSW 2006 Australia
Fax: (61) (2) 9351-6022
E-mail: j.brandmiller@staff.usyd.edu.au
Website:
   www.biochem.usyd.edu.au/~jennie/GI/glycemic
   _index.html

REGISTERED DIETITIANS

Registered Dietitians (RDs) are nutrition experts who provide nutritional assessment and guidance and support for people with heart disease. Check for the initials "RD" after the name to identify qualified dietitians who provide the highest standard of care to their clients. The glycemic index is part of their training, so all RDs should be able to help in applying the principles in this guide, but some dietitians do specialize in certain areas. If you want more detailed advice on the glycemic index, when you make your appointment just ask the dietitian whether this is a specialty.

Dietitians work in hospitals and often run their own private practices as well. For a list of dietitians in your area, call the American Dietetic Association (ADA) Consumer Nutrition Hotline (1-800-366-1655) or visit ADA's home page at the address below. You can also check the Yellow Pages under "Dietitians."

The American Dietetic Association
216 West Jackson Boulevard
Chicago, IL 60606
Phone: 1-800-877-1600
Fax: 1-312-899-1979
Web site: www.eatright.org

PRIMARY CARE PHYSICIANS

If you have heart disease or think you may have it, keep in close contact with your primary care physician or heart specialist.

WEIGHT LOSS ORGANIZATIONS

To help you lose weight, check the Yellow Pages under "Weight Control Services." Be aware, however, that not all weight loss organizations are reputable. Check with your physician to make sure the group you'd like to join can help you lose weight safely.

DIABETES ORGANIZATIONS

Extra weight can often make a diabetic condition worse. For more information about living with and controlling your diabetes, contact the following:

The American Diabetes Association
1660 Duke Street
Alexandria, VA 22314
Phone: 1-800-ADA-DISC (1-800-232-3472)
Web site: www.diabetes.org

Canadian Diabetes Association National Office
15 Toronto Street Suite #800
Toronto, ON M5C 2E3
Phone: 1-800-BANTING (1-800-226-8464) or 1-416-363-3373
Web site: www.diabetes.ca

NATURAL OVENS (ORDERING INFORMATION)

Natural Ovens of Manitowoc
4300 County Trunk CR
PO Box 730
Manitowoc, WI 54221-073
Telephone: 1-800-772-0730
Fax: 1-920-758-2594
Web site: www.naturalovens.com

ABOUT THE AUTHORS

Heather Gilbertson, B. Sc., Grad. Dip. Diet., Grad. Cert. Diab. Ed., APD, an accredited practicing dietitian and diabetes educator, has extensive experience in diabetes management in children and adolescents and has researched the effect of low glycemic index and measured carbohydrate diets in children with diabetes. She currently works at the Women's and Children's Health Care Network, Royal Children's Hospital Campus, Melbourne and conducts a private practice in the Macedon Ranges, Victoria, Australia.

Jennie Brand-Miller, Ph.D., Associate Professor of Human Nutrition in the Human Nutrition Unit, Department of Biochemistry, University of Sydney, Australia, is a world authority on the glycemic index of foods. She received her B.Sc. (1975) and Ph.D. (1979) degrees from the Department of Food Science and Technology at the University of New South Wales, Australia. She is the editor of the *Proceedings of the Nutrition Society of Australia* and a member of the Scientific Consultative Committee of the Australian Nutrition Foundation. She has written more than 200 research papers, including 60 on the glycemic index of foods. A co-author of *The Glucose Revolution* and all the titles in *The Glucose Revolution Pocket Guide* series, she lives in Sydney, Australia. Her most recent book is *The Glucose Revolution Life Plan*.

Kaye Foster-Powell, B. Sc., M.Nutr. & Diet, is an accredited practicing dietitian-nutritionist. A graduate of the University of Sydney (B.Sc., 1987; Master of Nutrition and Dietetics, 1994), she has extensive experience in diabetes management and has completed lengthy research on practical applications of the glycemic index. She is the senior dietitian at Wentworth Area Diabetes Service and conducts a private practice in the Blue Mountains, New South Wales. Her most recent book is *The Glucose Revolution Life Plan*.

Thomas M.S. Wolever, M.D., Ph.D., another of the world's leading researchers of the glycemic index, is Professor in the Department of Nutritional Sciences, University of Toronto, and a member of the Division of Endocrinology and Metabolism, St. Michael's Hospital, Toronto. He is a graduate of Oxford University (B.A., M.A., M.B., B. Ch., M.Sc., and D.M.) in the United Kingdom. He received his Ph.D. at the University of Toronto. His research since 1980 has focused on the glycemic index of foods and the prevention of type 2 diabetes. A co-author of *The Glucose Revolution* and all the titles in *The Glucose Revolution Pocket Guide* series, he lives in Toronto, Canada.

Johanna Burani, M.S., R.D., C.D.E., is a registered dietitian and certified diabetes educator with more than 11 years experience in nutritional counseling. She specializes in designing individual meal plans based on low G.I. food choices. The adapter of *The Glucose Revolution* and the co-adapter, with Linda Rao, of all the titles in *The Glucose Revolution Pocket Guide* series, she is the author of seven books and professional manuals, and lives in Mendham,

New Jersey. Her most recent book is *The Glucose Revolution Life Plan*.

Linda Rao, M.Ed., a freelance writer and editor, has been writing and researching health topics for the past 12 years. Her work has appeared in several national publications, including *Prevention*, *Cooking Light*, and *USA Today*. She serves as a contributing editor for *Prevention* magazine and is the co-adapter, with Johanna Burani, of all the titles in *The Glucose Revolution Pocket Guide* series. She lives in Allentown, Pennsylvania.

ACKNOWLEDGMENTS

We would like to acknowledge the extraordinary efforts of Johanna Burani and Linda Rao, who adapted this book—and the other books in *The Glucose Revolution Pocket Guide* series—for North American readers. Together they have worked to ensure that every piece of information is accurate and appropriate for readers in the U.S. and Canada.

For more information about *The Glucose Revolution, The Glucose Revolution Life Plan,* and *The Glucose Revolution Pocket Guides,* visit **www.glucoserevolution.com**

The Glucose Revolution begins here . . .

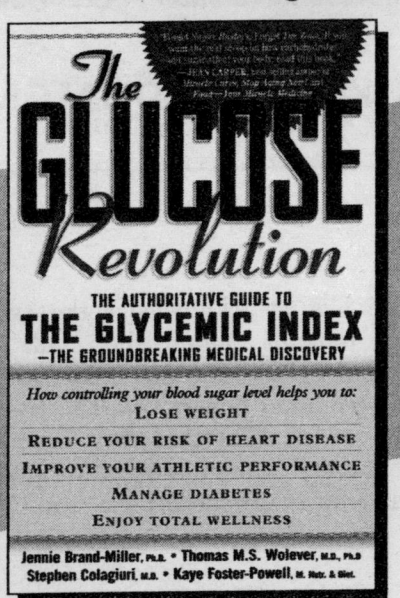

THE GLUCOSE REVOLUTION
THE AUTHORITATIVE GUIDE TO THE GLYCEMIC INDEX— THE GROUNDBREAKING MEDICAL DISCOVERY

NATIONAL BESTSELLER!

"Forget *Sugar Busters*. Forget *The Zone*. If you want the real scoop on how carbohydrates and sugar affect your body, read this book by the world's leading researchers on the subject. It's the authoritative, last word on choosing foods to control your blood sugar."

—JEAN CARPER, best-selling author of *Miracle Brain, Miracle Cures, Stop Aging Now!* and *Food—Your Miracle Medicine*

ISBN 1-56924-660-2 • $14.95

... and continues with these other *Glucose Revolution Pocket Guides*

The Glucose Revolution Pocket Guide to
LOSING WEIGHT

Eat yourself slim with low glycemic index foods

Not all foods are created equal when it comes to losing weight. The latest medical research shows that carbohydrates with a low glycemic index have special advantages because they fill you up and keep you satisfied longer. This pocket guide will help you eat yourself slim with low glycemic index foods and show you how low glycemic index foods make sustained weight loss possible. This guide also includes a 7-day low glycemic index plan for losing weight, G.I. success stories, and the glycemic index and fat and carbohydrate content of more than 300 foods and drinks.
ISBN 1-56924-677-7 • $4.95

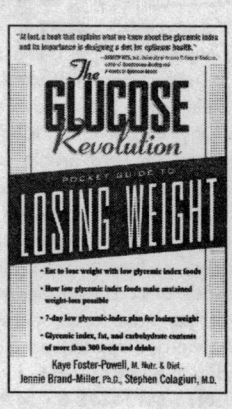

The Glucose Revolution Pocket Guide to
SPORTS NUTRITION

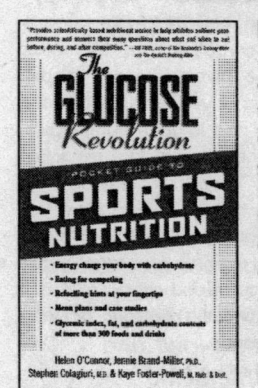

Eat to compete better than ever before.

Serious athletes and weekend warriors can gain a winning edge by manipulating the glycemic index of their diets. Now this at-a-glance guide shows how to use the glycemic index to boost athletic performance, enhance stamina, and prevent fatigue. Subjects covered include energy charging with carbohydrates, eating for competing, refueling hints, menu plans and case studies, and the glycemic index, fat and carbohydrate content of more than 300 foods and drinks.
ISBN 1-56924-676-9 • $4.95

The Glucose Revolution Pocket Guide to
DIABETES

Help control your diabetes with low glycemic index foods

Based on the most up-to-date information about carbohydrates, this basic guide to the glycemic index and diabetes allows people with type 1 and type 2 diabetes to make more informed choices about their diets. Topics covered include why many traditionally "taboo" foods don't cause the unfavorable effects on blood sugar levels they were believed to have, and why diets based on low G.I. foods improve blood sugar control. Also covered are how to include more of the right kinds of carbohydrates in your diet, the optimum diet for people with diabetes, practical hints for meal preparation and tips to help make the glycemic index work throughout the day, a week of low G.I. menus, G.I. success stories, and more.

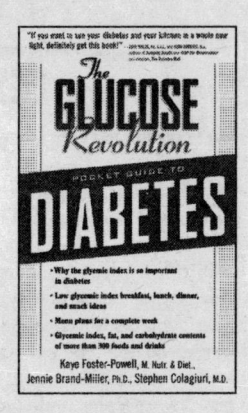

ISBN 1-56924-675-0 • $4.95

The Glucose Revolution Pocket Guide to
SUGAR AND ENERGY

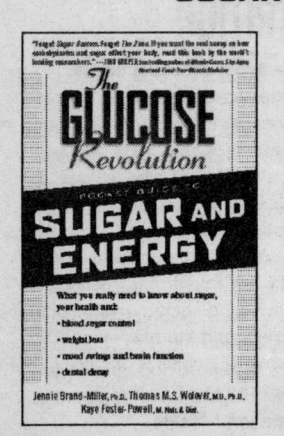

Sugar's off the black list—find out why

Based on the most up-to-date information about carbohydrates, this basic guide to the glycemic index dispels many common myths about sugar and why it's high time to get rid of the guilt. With evidence showing that restricting refined sugar in your diet may do more harm than good, the authors show you how to intelligently give in to your sugar cravings and regulate your sugar intake to control your blood sugar level and lose weight, with the glycemic index for nearly 150 foods.

ISBN 1-56924-641-6 • $4.95

The Glucose Revolution Pocket Guide to
THE TOP 100 LOW GLYCEMIC FOODS

The best of the best in low glycemic index foods

The slow digestion and gradual rise and fall in blood sugar levels after a food with a low glycemic index has benefits for many people. Today we know the glycemic index of hundreds of different generic and name-brand foods, which have been tested following a standardized method. Now *The Top 100 Low Glycemic Foods* makes it easy to enjoy those slowly digested carbohydrates every day for better blood sugar control, weight loss, a healthy heart, and peak athletic performance.

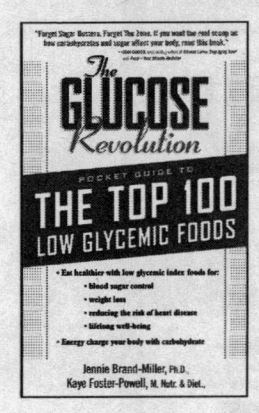

ISBN 1-56924-678-5 • $4.95

The Glucose Revolution Pocket Guide to
CHILDREN WITH TYPE 1 DIABETES

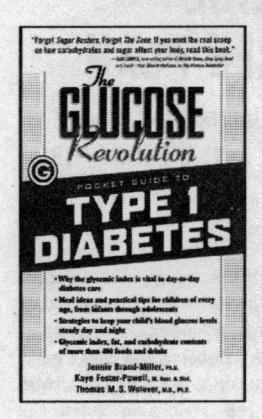

Discover How the Glycemic Index Can Be a Vital Part of Day-to-Day Diabetes Care

People with diabetes have been among the first to recognize the health benefits of the glycemic index (G.I.). Now the world's leading authorities on the G.I. explain how to use the G.I. in the daily management of Type 1 diabetes. Packed with useful information, this guide covers the benefits of knowing the G.I. values of foods, age-specific information for babies, toddlers, pre-schoolers, school-age children, and teenagers; meal ideas for breakfast, lunch, dinner, desserts, snacks, and parties; strategies to keep blood glucose levels steady day and night and much more.

ISBN 1-56924-638-6 • $4.95

THE GLUCOSE REVOLUTION LIFE PLAN

DISCOVER HOW TO MAKE THE GLYCEMIC INDEX—THE MOST SIGNIFICANT DIETARY FINDING OF THE LAST 25 YEARS—THE FOUNDATION FOR A LIFETIME OF HEALTHY EATING

Both an introduction to the benefits of low-G.I. foods and an essential source for those already familiar with the concept, *The Glucose Revolution Life Plan* presents the glycemic index within the context of today's full nutrition picture. With the glycemic index as its starting point, it gives readers clear guidelines for choosing the diet that is right for them. With the most authoritative, up-to-date and complete table of G.I. values published anywhere, *The Glucose Revolution Life Plan* makes the glycemic index accessible and useful to more readers than ever before.

ISBN 1-56924-609-2 • $18.95

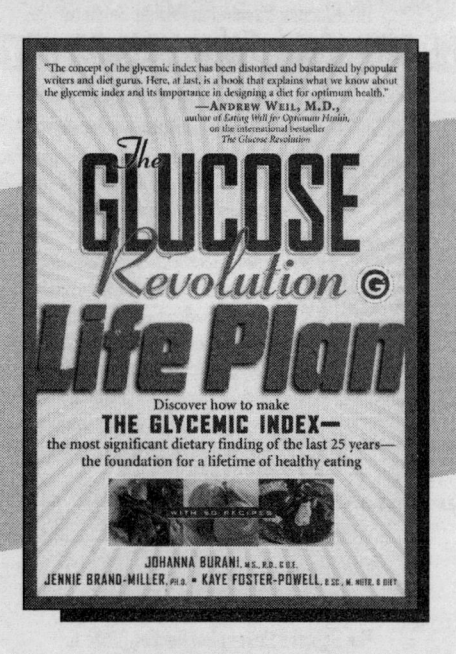